CHRISTINE CRAGGS-HINTON, mother of three, followed a career in the Civil Service until, in 1991, she developed fibromyalgia, a chronic pain condition. Christine took up writing for therapeutic reasons and has, in the past few years, produced *Living with Fibromyalgia, The Fibromyalgia Healing Diet, The Chronic Fatigue Healing Diet, Coping with Polycystic Ovary Syndrome* and *Coping with Gout* (all published by Sheldon Press). She also writes for the Fibromyalgia Association UK and the related *FaMily* magazine. In recent years she has become interested in fiction writing, too.

Overcoming Common Problems Series

Selected titles
A full list of titles is available from Sheldon Press,
36 Causton Street, London SW1P 4ST, and on our website at
www.sheldonpress.co.uk

Assertiveness: Step by Step
Dr Windy Dryden and Daniel Constantinou

The Assertiveness Handbook
Mary Hartley

Breaking Free
Carolyn Ainscough and Kay Toon

Calm Down
Paul Hauck

The Candida Diet Book
Karen Brody

Cataract: What You Need to Know
Mark Watts

The Chronic Fatigue Healing Diet
Christine Craggs-Hinton

Cider Vinegar
Margaret Hills

Comfort for Depression
Janet Horwood

Confidence Works
Gladeana McMahon

Coping Successfully with Irritable Bowel
Rosemary Nicol

Coping Successfully with Pain
Neville Shone

Coping Successfully with Panic Attacks
Shirley Trickett

Coping Successfully with Period Problems
Mary-Claire Mason

Coping Successfully with Prostate Cancer
Dr Tom Smith

Coping Successfully with Ulcerative Colitis
Peter Cartwright

Coping Successfully with Your Hiatus Hernia
Dr Tom Smith

Coping with a Stressed Nervous System
Dr Kenneth Hambly and Alice Muir

Coping with Alopecia
Dr Nigel Hunt and Dr Sue McHale

Coping with Anxiety and Depression
Shirley Trickett

Coping with Blushing
Dr Robert Edelmann

Coping with Bowel Cancer
Dr Tom Smith

Coping with Brain Injury
Maggie Rich

Coping with Candida
Shirley Trickett

Coping with Chemotherapy
Dr Terry Priestman

Coping with Childhood Allergies
Jill Eckersley

Coping with Childhood Asthma
Jill Eckersley

Coping with Chronic Fatigue
Trudie Chalder

Coping with Coeliac Disease
Karen Brody

Coping with Cystitis
Caroline Clayton

Coping with Depression and Elation
Patrick McKeon

Coping with Down's Syndrome
Fiona Marshall

Coping with Dyspraxia
Jill Eckersley

Coping with Eczema
Dr Robert Youngson

Coping with Endometriosis
Jo Mears

Coping with Epilepsy
Fiona Marshall and
Dr Pamela Crawford

Coping with Fibroids
Mary-Claire Mason

Coping with Gout
Christine Craggs-Hinton

Coping with Heartburn and Reflux
Dr Tom Smith

Coping with Incontinence
Dr Joan Gomez

Overcoming Common Problems Series

Coping with Long-Term Illness
Barbara Baker

Coping with Macular Degeneration
Dr Patricia Gilbert

Coping with the Menopause
Janet Horwood

Coping with a Mid-life Crisis
Derek Milne

Coping with Polycystic Ovary Syndrome
Christine Craggs-Hinton

Coping with Postnatal Depression
Sandra L. Wheatley

Coping with SAD
Fiona Marshall and Peter Cheevers

Coping with Snoring and Sleep Apnoea
Jill Eckersley

Coping with Strokes
Dr Tom Smith

Coping with Suicide
Maggie Helen

Coping with Thyroid Problems
Dr Joan Gomez

Curing Arthritis – The Drug-Free Way
Margaret Hills

Curing Arthritis Diet Book
Margaret Hills

Curing Arthritis Exercise Book
Margaret Hills and Janet Horwood

Depression
Paul Hauck

Depression at Work
Vicky Maud

Depressive Illness
Dr Tim Cantopher

Eating Disorders and Body Image
Christine Craggs-Hinton

Eating for a Healthy Heart
Robert Povey, Jacqui Morrell and Rachel Povey

Effortless Exercise
Dr Caroline Shreeve

Fertility
Julie Reid

The Fibromyalgia Healing Diet
Christine Craggs-Hinton

Free Your Life from Fear
Jenny Hare

Getting a Good Night's Sleep
Fiona Johnston

Heal the Hurt: How to Forgive and Move On
Dr Ann Macaskill

Heart Attacks – Prevent and Survive
Dr Tom Smith

Help Your Child Get Fit Not Fat
Jan Hurst and Sue Hubberstey

Helping Children Cope with Anxiety
Jill Eckersley

Helping Children Cope with Change and Loss
Rosemary Wells

Helping Children Get the Most from School
Sarah Lawson

How to Be Your Own Best Friend
Dr Paul Hauck

How to Beat Pain
Christine Craggs-Hinton

How to Cope with Bulimia
Dr Joan Gomez

How to Cope with Difficult People
Alan Houel and Christian Godefroy

How to Improve Your Confidence
Dr Kenneth Hambly

How to Keep Your Cholesterol in Check
Dr Robert Povey

How to Stick to a Diet
Deborah Steinberg and Dr Windy Dryden

How to Stop Worrying
Dr Frank Tallis

Hysterectomy
Suzie Hayman

The Irritable Bowel Diet Book
Rosemary Nicol

Is HRT Right for You?
Dr Anne MacGregor

Letting Go of Anxiety and Depression
Dr Windy Dryden

Lifting Depression the Balanced Way
Dr Lindsay Corrie

Living with Alzheimer's
Tom Smith

Living with Asperger Syndrome
Joan Gomez

Living with Asthma
Dr Robert Youngson

Living with Autism
Fiona Marshall

Overcoming Common Problems Series

Overcoming Common Problems

How to Beat Pain
Techniques that work

Christine Craggs-Hinton

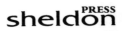

First published in Great Britain in 2005

Sheldon Press
36 Causton Street
London SW1P 4ST

The author and publisher have made every effort to ensure
that the external website and email addresses included in this book are correct
and up to date at the time of going to press. The author and publisher are
not responsible for the content, quality or continuing acessibility of the sites.

British Library Cataloguing-in-Publication Data

A catalogue record for this book is available from the British Library

ISBN 0–85969–945–5

1 3 5 7 9 10 8 6 4 2

Typeset by Deltatype Limited, Birkenhead, Merseyside
Printed in Great Britain by
Ashford Colour Press

Contents

Introduction

This book is for anyone who suffers from chronic pain – 'chronic' meaning pain or discomfort that has persisted intermittently or continuously for three months or more. Whether you are affected by repeated headaches, migraines, trigeminal neuralgia, post-herpetic neuralgia (the pain after shingles) or the pain of osteoarthritis, rheumatoid arthritis, osteoporosis, fibromyalgia, spondylitis, spinal stenosis, scoliosis, sciatica and so on, you should find a way out within these pages. The same applies for people with 'common back pain' – that is, pain where there is no specific diagnosis, caused by persistent muscle tension or strain.

The press often tells us that back pain alone is responsible for an estimated 60 million lost working days each year, costing the economy an annual £3 billion. What is never announced is the fact that chronic pain – in which back pain figures highly – is actually weakening the fabric of Western society, for the complications that come with it – sleep disturbance, anxiety, fear, moodiness, loss of confidence, depression and social isolation – can lead to unemployment, family disharmony, divorce and even bankruptcy.

The effect of my condition on my own family will always stay with me. It's almost 14 years since I became ill with fibromyalgia, and in the early years my muscles were in such distress that the weight of my arms on my shoulder muscles, and of my head on my neck and upper back muscles, caused intense pain. Normal actions like bending and reaching were out of the question and my husband had no choice but to take over the running of the house. He also had to wash me, brush my hair and feed me. I had no option but to spend the majority of my time lying down, convinced I had fallen victim to some terrible fatal disease. Yes, I know all about anxiety, fear, loss of confidence, depression and so on. It didn't help that I was drugged up to the eyeballs on prescribed medications, needing stronger and stronger dosages to achieve the same result.

Because I was no longer earning and my husband now my full-time carer, the children were suddenly without treats and family outings. I can hardly bear to think of them seeing their mother lying palely in bed every day ... As a result, they found it difficult to concentrate and their schoolwork suffered. One of my sons was about to start at a new school when I was at my worst. A clever boy, he just couldn't cope with my condition combined with the stress of new teachers, and a new routine, and constantly played truant, failing badly at his GCSEs – and all because of me. Or should I say, because of my pain. Thankfully, these days, I'm much more able to be there for my family after following the techniques outlined in this book, and for their part, my children learned resilience and understanding from that tough time, and are doing extremely well in their chosen professions.

I remember rallying emotionally after finally being given a diagnosis – even though I was to learn that, as far as conventional medicine was concerned, my condition was incurable. However, giving up hope of a magic 'cure' is sometimes no bad thing as it makes you explore other options and take more responsibility for your well-being. There is evidence to suggest that when chronic pain is diagnosed, people often find acceptance and resolution, and come to terms with what is happening in their lives. Many stop searching for that elusive cure, looking instead for therapeutic treatments that work best for them. In my case, it was the gentle exercise regime taught me by a rehabilitation physiotherapist that first got me out of bed. It slowly gave my muscles a degree of flexibility, began to loosen up my joints and gradually made it possible for me to sit up for an hour and a half at a time. I perform a daily exercise routine to this day. I am only too aware of the benefit it brings.

It is important that anyone with a chronic pain problem is offered referral to a pain-management programme – they exist in most areas. Such programmes are undoubtedly the best recent Health Service initiative regarding chronic pain, and many people return afterwards to far happier, more productive lives. Pain-management programmes are staffed by physiotherapists, psychologists, rheumatologists and GPs and are usually located in hospitals or doctors' surgeries. The two-week programme teaches stretching exercises, relaxation techniques and the most effective usage of medications. There is also a strong emphasis on 'cognitive behavioural therapy', where the individual is given guidance on tackling social situations, on working toward achievable goals, on better communicating their anxieties to the people around them and, all in all, on getting much more from their lives. My own referral to such a programme was one of the turning points for me.

Another turning point was starting to eat more healthily. I learnt from nutritionist friends that food is the finest medicine we can put into our bodies; and perhaps the best means of influencing overall health. They informed me about the need for nutritional supplements in dealing with chronic pain, explaining that where there is illness, the body is automatically deficient in certain vitamins and minerals. So, in order to fulfil my daily nutritional requirements, I began taking the recommended supplements as an adjunct to improving my diet. My energy levels rose quite quickly – then, as the months passed, I was delighted to be experiencing less pain.

When another friend introduced me to the concept of correct posture through the Alexander Technique, I was able to identify the massive levels of tension in my body – mainly because I was holding myself in such a poor way. I learnt to become aware of myself as a whole – my mind, body and spirit, for the Alexander Technique links the way in which our thought processes, emotions and feelings affect our bodies. It was after learning the most pain-free way to work at a computer that I began writing my first book, *Living with Fibromyalgia*.

From then on, I tried lots of different therapies and techniques, to varying effect. I was writing about them, too, giving advice to others coping with chronic pain in local and national newsletters. However, it was becoming increasingly clear that there are fundamental tools that enable people to start to climb out of their pit of pain and despair. To recap, these tools are:

- good nutrition for improvements on the inside
- the Alexander Technique for improved posture
- exercise for improved flexibility and strength.

It is only recently that I have come across a fourth tool. I became aware of the great benefits of trigger-point therapy – and soon realized that this was the missing link. I was given trigger-point injections in the early days of my illness, but as a trigger point is like a tiny rubber ball and difficult to hit with a needle, the injections were not particularly successful.

With my help, however, you will be able to locate your own

trigger points, for they exist in anyone with chronic pain. By using a special kind of self-applied massage that is described clearly in the first chapter, significant relief can come in just minutes. Less severe problems can be rectified in days. Long-standing chronic pain can be resolved in one to six months.

Although trigger-point therapy in itself is capable of dispelling a chronic pain situation, the problem is likely to recur if my other therapies are not taken on board. This book looks at several therapies which can boost quality of life, but in my opinion, exercise, good posture, optimum nutrition and trigger-point therapy make up an important four-pronged attack on pain. It is certainly working for me.

Note: The advice in this book is best followed with your doctor's approval. The author is not able to dispense medical advice independently, nor can she prescribe remedies or assume any responsibility for those who treat themselves without the consent of their doctor. As some nutritional supplements may interact with certain medications, and as they may adversely affect particular medical conditions, please consult your doctor before embarking upon a course.

1

Trigger-point therapy

Trigger points are tiny nodules in muscle fibres that send out 'referred' pain to different areas of the body. A word about 'referred' pain – I go into this further below, but as this is an important point with regard to understanding trigger points, I'd like to explain it a little now. Usually, with pain, you expect that the cause (or trigger) of the pain to be found on the exact spot that you feel the pain. But trigger points very often send pain to some other spot – they can literally 'trigger' pain elsewhere in the body. For example, a headache in the jaw may be caused by a trigger point in the neck. The fact that pain can be referred is one reason why trigger points have usually been missed by most people, including those working in conventional medicine.

How do trigger points start? Their development has many causes, including injury, muscle overuse, emotional stress, poor posture, poor general health and a co-existing health problem. Once fixed into a muscle, trigger points are often fiercely unwilling to give up their hold. Indeed, they are likely to spread from one muscle to another, causing not only chronic pain, but also a problem that may be difficult for medical professionals to diagnose.

Have you ever dreamt of finding a magic switch that could miraculously turn off your pain? It's a well-kept secret that there is such a switch – that tiny nodule in your muscle. To turn it off, it takes only the appliance of a simple massage technique, described later in this chapter. In some people the pain may vanish after only one short treatment, but on the whole it takes a little longer than that. Still, trigger-point therapy appears to be the briefest and most effective treatment available today. That the individual can carry out the therapy alone, within his or her four walls, is a terrific plus point – as is the fact that it incurs no cost, and you don't have to wait for an appointment.

You may, however, prefer to be treated by a skilled therapist. Trigger-point therapy has not yet been widely adopted in the UK, but some physiotherapy units are starting to offer it. Don't be too disappointed if you can't find a therapist in your area, though. The

1

technique is easy enough for most people to treat themselves.

Because I am keen to cover other valuable techniques in this book, I am able only to discuss trigger points in the main muscles of the head, neck and back. I recommend that you also purchase *The Trigger Point Therapy Workbook* (see 'Further reading') for more on other trigger points.

Trigger points: the mystery revealed

Many people with a pain problem have read that trigger-point therapy can be helpful, but have probably found no information as to exactly how it can be applied. It was the same with me. Then I read the 1999 edition of Travell and Simons' book *Myofascial Pain and Dysfunction: The Trigger Point Manual*, and considered it a revelation. I will therefore attempt, in this chapter, to describe for you the key points of trigger-point therapy, and to show you how to implement them yourself.

There are 696 muscles in the human body, and muscle tissue accounts for about 40 per cent of the body's total weight. Trigger points most commonly affect the muscles of the neck, shoulder girdle, low back and hip girdle. When trigger points are ignored as a possible cause of pain, they can remain active for many years – sometimes decades. Untreated trigger points result in muscle weakness and restricted movement. In addition, persistent pain invariably creates psychological problems such as anxiety, depression and loss of self-esteem.

According to the studies quoted by Travell and Simons, 85 per cent of pain-clinic patients experience pain that comes solely from trigger points, and trigger points are an element in a huge 93 per cent of cases. It can be seen, then, that trigger points feature highly in virtually all cases of chronic pain. It's an unfortunate fact, though, that many pain specialists are unaware that trigger points are likely to be involved in a pain problem. Some people are wrongly diagnosed with such incurable maladies as arthritis, disc degeneration or worn cartilage and are given a series of cortisone injections. Others may undergo invasive surgery such as vertebral fusion – and often to no avail. TENS machines, magnets, heated wheat bags and so on can reduce pain for a while, but make no difference at all in the long term. The patient is left with painkillers to depend on and little hope of being ultimately pain-free. We can only hope that the excellent work of Travell and Simons is soon brought to the wider world, and that the likely involvement of trigger points is considered early on in investigation and treatment.

What exactly is a trigger point?

A trigger point is a nodule-like knot within one of the many fibres in a muscle. Such a knot is capable also of occurring within the thin membranous sheath containing the muscle, although this is generally limited to where scar tissue is present. Trigger points are formally known as *myofascial trigger points* – *myo* meaning muscle and *fascia* meaning the membranous sheath. To the fingertips, trigger points may feel like a small bump, and may be as tiny as a pinhead or, in rare cases, as large as a thumb knuckle. If your fingertips are not particularly sensitive and you are wondering whether you will be able to locate your trigger points, don't worry – you will know when you have hit one because it will hurt!

All trigger points are tender on palpation (light finger pressure), but ones that are active cause an involuntary twitch or jerk from the pain (Vecchiet, 1990). From a doctor's perspective, the more intense the pain and the greater the twitch, the more likelihood there is of referred pain being present – that is, pain sent from the trigger point to a distant site (Hong, 1997). A person experiencing referred pain from one or more trigger points has 'myofascial pain syndrome', and it is believed that a great many more people suffer from this syndrome than doctors are currently aware.

It is important to note that a trigger point is not the same as a muscle spasm. A spasm is a violent contraction of the entire muscle, whereas a trigger point is a contraction of a small part of the muscle.

How a trigger point develops

Muscle contraction – the tensing and flexing of muscles – is made possible by the millions of microscopic components called *sarcomeres* that muscle fibres carry. Sarcomeres contract and release to pump blood through the capillaries that supply the muscle's needs. However, when sarcomeres become over-stimulated for reasons of stress, overuse and so on, they can stop being able to relax. As a consequence, blood flow in that region is greatly reduced and

3

oxygen deprivation and waste build-up occur. This is the beginning of a trigger point.

Immediately, the affected muscle fibre, unhappy about the development of the trigger point, sends out panic signals to the brain. The brain responds by telling the individual to rest the muscle. However, the unfortunate result of rest in this instance is that the muscle begins to shorten and become taut. The trigger points become amplified, and the affected muscle fibres become shortened and stringy. Full lengthening of the muscle is soon not possible, as a result of which there is restricted mobility. Muscle fatigue and decreased strength will naturally ensue from this situation.

Possible complications of trigger points

The muscles that have been shortened and made taut by trigger points often pinch neighbouring nerves – and when a nerve is pinched, the electrical impulses carried along that nerve cause numbness, tingling or stabbing in the areas the nerve serves. A pinched nerve in the upper back or neck will generally cause numbness, tingling or stabbing in the arms and hands. A pinched nerve in the lower back will generally cause the same sensations in the legs and feet.

A muscle affected by a trigger point is capable also of compressing an artery, reducing its blood flow and making a distant area feel cold. When this occurs in a particular neck muscle (the anterior scalene), the result can actually be a swollen wrist and hand. Trigger points in a particular calf muscle (the soleus) can obstruct the return of blood in a vein, causing a swollen ankle or foot.

The heart, blood vessels, respiratory system, skin, glands, and digestive system are controlled by the body's autonomic system (i.e. the body's unconscious nervous system which controls functions such as heartbeat and breathing). Trigger points on the smooth muscles of this system have been shown to cause such strange effects as nasal excretion, excessive salivation, blurred vision, excessive tearing, reddening of the eyes, a droopy eyelid, goose-bumps, dizziness and even emotional distress (Perle, 1995).

Referred pain

Active trigger points can send pain or discomfort to some other site, often quite far away. For example, pain down one leg is likely to be caused by a trigger point in the lower back or buttocks. The trigger point is the pain generator, but the majority of the pain is felt in distant sites.

Unfortunately, many hours can be spent rubbing areas that are painful. If you are very lucky, you can make the pain abate for a short while, but rubbing referred pain sites will never stop the pain in its tracks. The only way to stop referred pain is to tackle the source – the trigger point.

Referred pain from trigger points is thought to cause or greatly contribute to the following:

- back and neck pain
- headaches and migraine
- carpal tunnel pain
- tennis elbow
- frozen shoulder
- earache, the pain of sinus congestion, jaw pain, heartburn and a sore throat
- painful knees, knuckles, wrists, ankles, elbows, shoulders and hips
- sore feet and legs
- pelvic pain and pain during sexual intercourse
- pain in the ovaries, cervix, uterus, penis, testes, prostate, rectum and bladder.

Stiffness and pain in any joint is likely to be caused by trigger points in another region.

What does referred pain feel like?

Referred pain is often a deep oppressive ache that occurs at rest or on movement, or both. In some cases, especially when nerve pain is present, the pain can be excruciating, often described as searing or stabbing. There may also be tingling and numbness.

Active or sleeping trigger point?

Not all trigger points refer pain to other areas. The ones that do are termed 'active' and the ones that don't are known as 'sleeping' or 'latent'. When you push on a nodule in a muscle and it causes pain in the immediate area (around the trigger point), rather than sending pain to another area, you have found one that is sleeping.

Sleeping trigger points can arise after a sprain in some of the

5

fibres of a muscle. During the healing period, the trigger point is active and there is a painful taut band within the affected muscle. In most people, the sprain heals naturally in one to two weeks, deactivating the trigger point and removing the pain. There are a few people in whom the pain resolves but the taut band remains, and it is in this that a sleeping trigger point lurks.

A sleeping trigger point does not normally cause pain unless it is prodded or squeezed. Because a sleeping trigger point may make the muscle less willing to lengthen or relax, the muscle can be vulnerable to further injury – and it takes only a small injury to make a sleeping trigger point spring into life.

Satellite trigger points

When there are further muscles within the pain referral zone of an active trigger point – which is usually the case – another trigger point can easily develop. For example, if an individual felt pain from a trigger point in the shoulder, satellite trigger points could set up in the muscles in the arm and before long the person would be aware of discomfort in the arm as well.

Since the zone of trigger-point radiation can be extensive, trigger points are capable of cascading from one muscle to another, causing widespread chronic pain in some.

Do I have a trigger point?

Apart from locating a knot or nodule in a muscle, you'll know you have an active trigger point in the following ways:

- You will have pain somewhere.
- You may experience stiffness in a muscle or joint that has been overworked.
- There may be referred pain in the pain referral zone for the muscle affected (see the second part of this chapter for patterns of referred pain).
- You may be able to feel a taut band within the muscle.
- You may notice that a certain muscle is weaker than normal. A muscle with one or more trigger points will lose some of its strength.
- When you press on what you suspect is a trigger point, you are likely to feel pain or tingling in further areas. This is a dead give-away that you have a trigger point.

What causes trigger points?

The overuse and abuse of muscles is the main reason that trigger points develop. If a woman taps away at a keyboard all day and her wrists are not adequately supported, a trigger point may form in the muscles at the side of her neck (*scalenes*), causing pain in her wrist – pain that may be incorrectly diagnosed as carpal tunnel syndrome or repetitive strain injury (RSI). If a man continually tips boxes of fruit on to a conveyor belt, twisting in an awkward manner in the process, he may develop trigger points in the muscles of his middle back (*superficial spinal muscles*). The referred pain, though, may be felt in his hip and buttock. It can be seen, then, that repeating or maintaining an awkward body position for long periods can result in the development of trigger points.

Trigger points can also occur in the following conditions:

- Failing to take breaks when carrying out unusually heavy work.
- Being out of condition prior to embarking on heavy work.
- Failing to take sufficient breaks when performing repetitive work. In the workplace, it would make good sense for managers to allocate staff a variety of jobs so they are not using one set of muscles repeatedly.
- Sitting for a long time in a chair that dictates poor posture – for example, a car seat, beanbag or bucket seat.
- Working at a computer with an offset screen, so your head is constantly turned to one side.
- Carrying a heavy weight on one shoulder – for example, a schoolchild carrying lots of books in a shoulder bag.
- Muscle fatigue. Repetitive movement or loading beyond a certain point will fatigue a muscle and eventually cause trigger points.
- After damage to an area. Trigger points often result from the sudden wrenching movement of a whiplash injury, for instance. The person may avoid turning and tilting his or her head in the weeks following the injury, as a result of which the 'cascade effect' can arise (see 'Satellite trigger points' above, page 6).
- Failing to warm the muscles before vigorous activity. For example, a sprinter who neglects to perform the correct stretch procedures is in danger of creating trigger points in his calf muscles.

- During hot or cold weather. In extreme weather, the blood and lymph fluid flow to the muscles can be compromised. This affects the flow of the minerals required for muscle and nerve function.

- Prolonged tension in the shoulder muscles in someone who is very anxious and stressed. Carrying out heavy work or a prolonged activity when the muscles are already contracted through tension can result in the formation of trigger points.

- Nutritional deficiencies. A poor diet will create unhealthy muscle tissue with poorer regenerative powers that are susceptible to breakdown.

- Bone abnormalities such as unequal leg lengths. In this instance, the muscles have to compensate continuously and trigger points may eventually develop. Bone abnormalities can also take the form of short upper arms, an asymmetrical pelvis and a long metatarsal bone (specifically the second toe) in the foot. In rare cases, all the bones in one side of the body can be smaller than on the other side.

- Constrictive clothing. When someone wears very tight clothing, sustained compression of the muscles can result in trigger points. For example, there are such medical conditions as 'jeans-related buttock pain', 'bra-strap headache' (the headache being referred pain), and 'wallet sciatica' (where the tension around the pocket in which the wallet is kept causes pressure on the sciatic nerve).

What causes trigger points to persist?

There are many reasons why trigger points can maintain their hold. Here are the main ones.

When trigger points develop due to abnormalities in bone structure, they can be difficult to remove. Legs of a slightly different length, for example, can result in constant strain on a particular group of muscles, creating and maintaining trigger points in the legs, buttocks, back and neck. In the same way, when one side of the pelvis is smaller than the other, the pelvis will tilt on sitting. As a result, the spine will curve abnormally, placing an extra load on the back muscles and even the neck muscles. Happily, heel lifts can resolve the situation with different leg lengths – they have even been known to stop persistent headaches. Sitting with one buttock on a thin pad or cushion can help to remedy an uneven pelvis and a smaller bone structure on one side of the body. People with shorter upper arms than normal should use elbow supports while sitting, and choose chairs with higher arms. When the back and neck are better supported, trigger points should gradually disappear.

A staggering 25 per cent of the population are at risk of trigger points due to the effects of 'Morton's Foot'. The condition is characterized by the fact that the bones (metatarsals) of the second toe are longer than the bones of the big toes. However, this does not necessarily make the second toes longer than the big toes. To gauge the lengths of the bones in these toes, bend them backwards at their heads. Long second metatarsals cause uneven distribution of body weight on the feet, often giving rise to heavy calluses – the first on the sole, under the head of the second toe; the others along the edge of the big toe and the first and fifth toes. The feet compensate by turning the toes outward and the ankles inward and by flattening the arch. Because of instability in the ankle and frequent ankle sprains, trigger points can arise in the lower leg and foot. This condition is best treated by placing a thin circular pad under the head of the first metatarsal – the ball of the foot – in all your footwear. Feather the edge of each pad with scissors and stick them to the bottom of a pair of cushioned insoles before placing in a pair of shoes. The pad will make you walk with your feet pointed forward instead of out to the side. Your feet will no longer look quite so flat, and your ankles will no longer turn in as much. Furthermore, pain in the foot and lower leg should gradually ease.

Many people are unaware that the way they sit and move is constantly stressing the muscles and causing trigger points to form. By far the best way to improve your posture is to follow the Alexander Technique (see Chapter 2).

Inactivity is a great perpetuator of trigger-point pain. We tend to protect ourselves by keeping painful muscles immobile. However, this encourages them to stiffen and become weak. It also encourages satellite trigger points.

Repetitive movement – however small – can overload the muscles and cause trigger points to persist. For example, sitting at a computer keyboard all day doesn't seem to take much effort, but the small muscles of the hands and forearms are constantly active. At the same time, the larger muscles of the shoulders, upper back and neck are immobile but under continuous contraction to hold your head and arms in position. It is the same with many of the jobs in industry. If possible, vary your activities, in the workplace or at home.

Nutritional deficiencies can make it easy for trigger points to persist. Read my nutrition advice in Chapter 4.

Harmful substances may perpetuate trigger points, including nicotine, caffeine and alcohol. Smoking causes high levels of the toxic chemical cadmium in the body. With caffeine, some experts consider that four cups of coffee a day (or six cups of tea) are safe, but others believe it is nearer two cups of coffee (or three cups of tea). Try to cut out alcohol, or drink only very small amounts as, like nicotine and caffeine, it is toxic to the body and may prevent trigger-point deactivation.

A shortfall in the body of relative growth hormone has recently been suggested as playing a pivotal role in trigger-point development. Growth hormone is necessary for muscle repair and its secretion is related to deep sleep, which is frequently disturbed in people with pain. It can be seen, then, that a shortfall of this hormone may make trigger points linger.

Another condition that can cause trigger points to persist is hypothyroidism – an inadequacy in the amount of daily thyroid hormone production, the symptoms of which include muscle cramps, cold intolerance, weakness, stiffness, chronic fatigue and pain.

Hypoglycaemia – low blood-sugar levels – can make trigger points difficult to deactivate, too. The symptoms of hypoglycaemia are a fast heartbeat, shaking, sweating and increased anxiety. Emotional distress can cause blood-sugar levels to fall, as can eating a diet full of 'simple carbohydrates' including table sugar, and sugars in sweets, cakes, biscuits and sweetened cereals.

If you suffer from gout – where there are raised levels of uric acid in the blood – urate crystals will deposit in the joints and may perpetuate trigger points. Gout can even make trigger points more troublesome than they might otherwise be. This painful inflammatory condition affecting the joints can be eased by weight loss in those who are overweight. Cutting down on alcohol and binge drinking can also lower levels of uric acid and make trigger points easier to get rid of, as can eliminating red meat, seafood, asparagus, mushrooms, yeast, dried peas and beans, lentils, soy and spinach. Some medications keep uric acid levels raised, such as aspirin and water tablets for high blood pressure. Ask your doctor if you can try an alternative medication, then see if your trigger points respond better.

Continuing to wear tight, constrictive clothing also makes trigger points more likely to persist.

Misdiagnosis of trigger points

Trigger points and the referred pain they cause are not discussed in medical school, as a result of which wrong diagnoses can occur. Mistaken diagnoses include tendonitis, bursitis, a ligament injury, disc problems and even arthritis. Trigger points in some muscles of the low back and leg are capable of causing referred pain. When this pain is mistakenly diagnosed as disc displacement – whereby the vertebral disc or its nucleus presses on the sciatic nerve – surgery can be considered the best option. However, the failure rate of surgery for low-back pain is high, about 53 per cent of all L5–S1 disc surgeries failing to relieve the symptoms (Radin, 1987). In fact, it is not at all unusual for the patient to end up in worse shape than before the operation.

For as long as some doctors fail to recognize and treat myofascial trigger points, misdiagnosis will continue to occur. Many GPs and orthopaedic surgeons know nothing of trigger points, and, as trigger points don't show up on X-rays or scans, patients may be told there is nothing wrong with them and that nothing can be done.

When trigger points are not treated

Trigger points keep the muscles from relaxing completely. They can cause them to tire quickly, recover slowly from exertion and contract excessively when they work.

The moving parts of the body were intended to move freely and completely through a specific range of motion, but trigger points can prevent this. The affected muscles become ropy and feel tight and enlarged. As a result, the individual is less mobile. When the cascade effect occurs, pain is more widespread and chronic disability can ensue.

What are trigger-point injections?

When trigger-point injections effectively penetrate that nodule in the muscle, they can reduce pain enough to allow the person to exercise the muscle gently and so make it less likely that the trigger point will

11

reappear. The injection comprises a low dose of local anaesthetic, which makes the trigger point relax, mixed with a low dose of steroid, which helps to reduce any post-injection soreness. However, not only is the trigger-point nodule generally very small – no larger than a pinhead in many instances – but it also has the consistency of a hard rubber ball, and tends to make the needle bounce off it or push it aside. Moreover, the nodule may be buried deep in the muscle and difficult to find. The use of electromyogram (EMG) guidance to locate trigger points and ensure they are successfully penetrated with the needle is the best option, but this type of treatment is not always on offer.

Passive stretching of the muscle immediately after the injection can be greatly beneficial. This type of stretching is carried out by the doctor or nurse, who gently moves the area of the body concerned through a range of motion. When passive stretching does not take place, the therapeutic effects of the injection are less.

Despite the steroid content of the injection, post-injection soreness occasionally occurs. There is also a risk – although minimal – of the doctor or anaesthetist accidentally damaging a blood vessel, a nerve or even a vital organ. A far more frequent error is injecting into a tender area or referred pain zone instead of a trigger point. Injecting into a tense, fibrous band that is not a true trigger point can irritate the surrounding tissue and make things worse.

Trigger-point injections are most beneficial when trigger points are fairly new; of course, whether your doctor will offer them so early is an entirely different matter. A chronic pain condition will generally require a series of injections as the problem is likely to be deeply entrenched. If you are fortunate enough to have a doctor who will refer you for injections, you then need to be fortunate enough to be treated by an anaesthetist who is skilled at successfully injecting trigger points.

Nowadays, some anaesthetists will consider using Botox A (Botulinum Toxin A) injections, especially where trigger-point injections have failed. You have no doubt heard of botox with regard to its being a deadly poison (in much larger doses) and a cosmetic anti-wrinkle substance . . . Well, it can also be of help to contracted muscle fibres. It works by preventing the motor-nerve impulses from reaching the injected fibre. Instead, it binds irreversibly to specific receptors, causing muscle relaxation that lasts for up to three months. In some cases, new receptors are then created, enabling muscle tone to return slowly. Other people may need further botox injections at intervals of three to six months.

The most common side-effects of botox injections are headache, slight bruising, flu-like symptoms and nausea. There may also be redness at the injection site and weakness of the muscle injected. The long-term effects of repeated botox injections are not known.

What is the spray-and-stretch technique?

The spray-and-stretch technique also demands care to obtain the required effect – that of relaxing the muscle out of its contraction. For that reason, the treatment should be carried out by a skilled therapist. The therapist will desensitize the skin overlaying the trigger point by spraying on a vaporizing coolant or laying ice on it for a few seconds. Because it is important that the underlying muscle is not chilled, the therapist will work quickly – cooling the muscle itself would prevent the stretch. The skin is now reheated by warm moist packs, after which the therapist gently moves the body through the complete range of motion without the use of force, which can strain the muscle's attachments. Trigger points generally react to stretching with a defensive tightening. By using the spray-and-stretch technique, the muscle can be lengthened without resistance. This method is carried out quite frequently in the USA, but less often in the UK.

The muscle-energy technique

It is possible for a therapist to deactivate a trigger point by applying firm pressure with a finger or thumb for 3–5 minutes. This literally squeezes the blood out of the tissues, depriving the trigger point temporarily of oxygen and so allowing it to relax. This technique – *ischemic compression* – is currently not often undertaken in the UK.

Carrying out this technique yourself can be difficult, and is not recommended. To apply pressure for a sustained period on an area that is painful already can cause more pain than is tolerable, and it can be tiring on the hands, arms and shoulders. Many of the massage therapists who use this technique experience constant pain in their arms and hands and end up retiring early from their jobs.

It is important, then, that your trigger points are released safely. Don't risk ending up with more problems than you started with.

13

The deep stroking massage

Experts believe that the safest and most effective method of deactivating trigger points is the deep stroking massage. With this technique, the muscle's attachments are not in jeopardy as they can be with the spray-and-stretch technique, and there is no risk of accidental damage as can occur with trigger-point injections. Moreover, it has a much better success rate.

Self-massage

While I feel bound to recommend professional trigger-point massage first and foremost, I have to say that combining it with self-treatment can improve its efficacy enormously. If you opt for skilled treatment and are treating yourself at home as well, be sure to inform the therapist concerned. At the end of the session, it would be useful for you to be shown the location of the primary and satellite trigger points identified by the therapist. You can then work on them yourself between appointments.

Unfortunately, some people may be unable to find a therapist who is skilled at trigger-point therapy and will have no choice but to self-treat – which is where this book comes in. Others will prefer to try out the massages at home first of all.

The benefits of self-massage include the following:

- You don't have to pay a therapist.
- You don't have to wait for an appointment.
- You don't have to spend time and money travelling to and from an appointment.
- You can treat yourself whenever you need it.
- You are likely to have a feeling about whether or not a particular treatment is working.
- To know you are helping yourself gives a sense of achievement.

Does trigger-point massage hurt?

Because the trigger point is, in most people, very painful in itself, working it is bound to cause pain. However, many people say it's a pleasant kind of pain, not at a level that would cause you to tense up. The electrical impulses you may feel as you massage a trigger point are neurological messages that are disrupting the feedback loop

14

perpetuating the trigger point. Healing begins as a result of this disruption. Don't be alarmed if you don't feel electrical impulses, though. If you are carrying out the massage properly, the trigger point will begin to heal.

It is important that you don't massage too heartily and too frequently, or you are likely to cause yourself more pain. Being too eager can not only bruise the skin, it can also bruise the deeper tissues such as the muscles and nerves. Working vigorously on several trigger points in one session can even cause dizziness and nausea. It often takes trial and error to discover how much pressure is required.

I would strongly advise that at first you tackle one trigger point at once, and then monitor the results. Also, it is best to work on your worst trigger points first and gradually come to the less painful ones.

How long will it take to get rid of my pain?

Trigger points that have been active for a number of years will have made pathways into the nervous system that reinforce and perpetuate the pain. It can take quite a long time to resolve this. Even then, it is not reasonable to expect that the trigger points will never come back – but now you should be able to keep on top of the problem.

When pain is still fairly new, trigger-point massage can get rid of it very quickly – usually in two or three days. It is often the same with pain that is localized – in the jaw, for example. Exactly how long a pain problem will take to resolve depends on the individual. Much depends on your ability to determine which is referred pain and which is the trigger point.

The importance of massaging the right spot

Attacking the pain and ignoring its cause does no good at all. You may feel you should be massaging the back of your shoulder because that is where the pain is, when in fact the trigger points responsible are in your neck. Massaging the back of your shoulder may ease the pain for a short while, but will do nothing to deactivate the trigger points. In order to find the accountable trigger points, it is important to become acquainted with patterns of referred pain. To find out where referred pain might be, look at my explanations further on, under the headings: 'Head and neck pain', page 19; 'Face and jaw

15

pain', page 28; 'Shoulder and upper-back pain', page 30; and 'Mid- and low-back pain', page 33.

The best way to find a trigger point is to feel about until you hit that spot of supreme tenderness. If you are not able to locate the tiny nodule, don't be disheartened. The nodule is at the centre of that area of tenderness, and this is where the massage should be applied.

The massage technique

The best way to encourage a trigger point to relax is to give a brief massage across the trigger-point nodule – or if you can't feel the nodule, across that area of extreme tenderness – lasting no more than 15–20 seconds. The massage should be in the form of short 1–1½-inch (3–4-cm) strokes in one direction only, done at the rate of approximately one stroke per second. This action enables you to push out blood and lymph fluid – the lymph fluid containing accumulated waste products from the continuous contraction of the fibres of the muscle. It is important, also, to slide with the skin, rather than over the skin. This encourages the membranous sheath of tissue that encloses the muscle to loosen up, for its tightness is sometimes part of the problem. Indeed, this thin sheath is occasionally the spot in which a trigger point lurks.

Try to make the strokes gradually deeper and deeper, pressing the nodule against the underlying bone. When you release your fingers (or knuckle, thumb or tool) after each stroke, fresh blood will flood into the area, carrying with it the revitalizing oxygen and nutrients of which it was previously starved. There is no particular direction in which you should stroke.

The level of pressure will depend on the area you are treating. For example, the muscles of the back require more pressure than the muscles of the forearm. The pressure should be midway between painful and pleasurable – it 'hurts so good'. If the sensations decrease, press harder. If that fails to bring the desired effect, you are likely to have slipped off the nodule and should try to relocate it.

If you have one or more trigger points that are far more painful than pleasurable to work, don't avoid doing so. You now have the knowledge to get rid of your pain. It would be a shame not to use it. Brave the pain for an initial deep stroke, then wait for ten seconds before continuing. This gives the endorphins, your body's natural painkillers, time to start flowing, enabling the remaining strokes to

16

be rather less painful. Being overly gentle is no good either. The stroke must be deep to release the knotted tissues. In other words, you have to cause yourself a certain amount of pain to be pain-free in the end.

When the technique is performed 6–12 times a day, the trigger point should release, upon which the referred pain will disappear. If the treatment fails, it may be because you are either being too aggressive or working on the wrong spot.

The following points outline the basics of the deep stroking technique:

- Make the strokes gentle, but work as deeply as you can, pressing the trigger point against bone.
- Use short strokes – each stroke being no more than 4 cm (1 ins) long.
- Stroke right across the trigger-point nodule, from one side to the other.
- Stroke in one direction only – the direction that feels most comfortable.
- Work no faster than one stroke per second.
- Whether you are using a fingertip, thumb, knuckle or tool, slide it with the skin rather than over the skin.
- Don't forget to remove your finger after each stroke, to allow fresh blood to flow into the area.
- Massage each trigger point between six and 12 times, and no more.
- The whole treatment on one trigger point should last for only 12–15 seconds.
- To save your hands, it is recommended that you use some kind of tool (see page 18, 'Using a massage tool').

Keeping your hands from injury during massage

Maximum penetration with the minimum of effort and strain is the aim for good trigger-point massage. If you wish to use your fingertips, it is essential that fingernails are cut to the quick. If you use the pads of your fingers you will reap little reward, as insufficient energy can be applied in this way. You will also tire far more quickly than if you were using your fingertips.

To safeguard hands from injury, support them in the following ways:

When *using your fingers for massage*, hold your hands at right angles to each other, the supporting hand covering the nails of the massaging fingers. Keep the wrist, hand and fingers straight and as relaxed as you can, and make the supporting hand help to move the fingertips of the tool hand. When using your thumb as a massage tool, keep it pressed close to the fingers as a means of support.

If you want to try *using your knuckles for massage*, you should use the joints mid-way along your fingers as the tool. The knuckles on your hand should be kept as straight as possible to transfer energy efficiently from your elbow, and your supporting hand should be held at right-angles to the other. This method of massage is less precise than the finger-stroke massage. If you are unwilling to cut your nails, however, you might want to opt for it.

Using a massage tool

There are a few massage tools on the market that will save your hands and allow you to reach otherwise inaccessible places. The leverage they give even boosts your strength. The best tools are probably the ones known as the Thera Cane, basically a J-shaped implement, and the Backnobber, which is the shape of a large S. Massage tools can be found in disability shops, physiotherapy suites and over the internet. (See 'Useful addresses'.) However, the majority of muscles can be worked by using a simple ball. For example, hanging a tennis ball in a sock over your shoulder and pressing yourself against a wall will, once you move yourself into the right position, allow for manipulation of anywhere on the back. Small high-bounce rubber balls are great for getting deep into the tissues, and using a ball against a wall eliminates the risk of hurting your hands. Just make sure you don't press the ball too deeply at first. Take it steadily and let your body tell you how much pressure to bring to bear.

Keep at it!

It's not enough to perform the technique a couple of times a week. Good results can be obtained only if you persist – after all, it takes only 15–20 seconds to carry out the massage on one trigger point, and you need only do 6–12 strokes at a time. If the first treatment causes bruising or the feeling that you have bruised yourself, don't give up. Wait until the bruising subsides, then use less pressure on your next treatment.

When you start to experience relief, you may want to drop one or two sessions of treatment and add one of the less painful trigger points to your regime. Don't be tempted to stop treatments in any one area as soon as the referred pain ceases, however. You may merely have lulled the trigger point into a sleeping condition, leaving it to be reactivated by the smallest of strains. For as long as the trigger point hurts when you press on it, you still have a problem.

Try to massage your trigger points shortly after getting up in the morning and just before going to bed at night – and several times during the day. If referred pain wakes you up during the night, work once more on the trigger point(s) responsible. It should give you enough relief to get back off to sleep.

Make your own pain chart

When you use the deep stroking technique, you will begin to recognize the best ways to get rid of pain in particular areas. For instance, you may find that using a massage tool worked better on that trigger point in your low back than anything else. It's important, then, to make your observations in writing. If you are anything like me, memory alone will not suffice.

The limitations of this book

Because I want to discuss the four major factors that can eradicate chronic pain, there are not enough pages in this book for me to describe every possible trigger-point site in the body. For that reason, I have chosen to discuss trigger points in the head, neck, shoulder and upper and lower back as being the most common areas where trigger points may be found. My hope is that you will become so skilled at locating trigger points here that you will be able to work on them with success in further areas.

Head and neck pain

Trigger points can cause a vast array of referred pain problems in the head and neck, including headache, migraine, earache, sinus pain, stiff neck, sore throat, eye pain and jaw pain. They can even cause

19

reddened eyes, a chronic cough, stuffiness in the ears, hypersensitive teeth, dizziness and balance problems. We all know that headaches are often provoked by a bad coughing attack, a hangover, overexertion, a viral infection, emotional stress, etc. – what occurs, in fact, is that a sleeping trigger point is activated by one of these processes.

The sternocleidomastoid

Lying at the front of the neck, toward the sides, the sternocleidomastoid attaches to the breastbone (sternum), the collarbone (clavicle) and the bony plate behind the ear (the mastoid process). Its main function is to turn the head to the opposite side. This muscle is rarely given the time of day, however – after all, you don't usually feel pain in the front of your neck. It would be wise to familiarize yourself with this muscle, for trigger points in the sternocleidomastoid can send out a great deal of pain.

The signature of trigger points in the sternocleidomastoid, sternal (frontmost) branch (Figure 1, 1a), is the frontal headache. Trigger points in this branch of the muscle can also cause referred pain in the eye, behind the ear, in the breastbone, in the jaw, over the eye, on top of the head and at the side of the face, the latter mimicking trigeminal neuralgia. It can also cause tongue pain on swallowing and will tend to perpetuate trigger points in the jaw muscles. Other problems are visual disturbances such as blurred or double vision, twitches in the muscle surrounding the eye, a drooping eyelid and runny nose. Trigger points in this muscle can also cause a cold sweat on the forehead, excess mucus in the sinuses and in the nasal cavities and throat, chronic cough and continual hay fever or cold symptoms. Very painful trigger points here can re-create or accentuate a frontal headache when the trigger point is pressed.

Trigger points in the clavicular branch of the sternocleidomastoid (Figure 1, 1b) can cause earache, toothache in the back molars and a frontal headache on the opposite side to the trigger point. Trigger points in this branch can also cause dizziness, nausea, fainting and even hearing loss on the same side as the trigger point.

As you can see from the diagrams, the sternal branch of the sternocleidomastoid lies in front of the clavicular branch. It is possible to take the sternal branch between your fingers and thumb, pull it aside and feel the clavicular branch behind it. Start behind

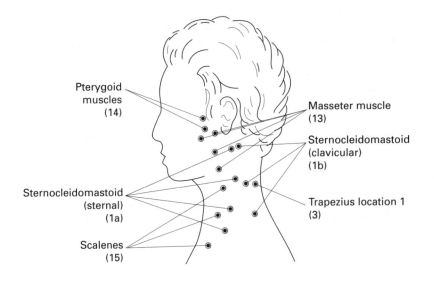

Pterygoid
muscles
(14)

Masseter muscle
(13)

Sternocleidomastoid
(clavicular)
(1b)

Sternocleidomastoid
(sternal)
(1a)

Trapezius location 1
(3)

Scalenes
(15)

Figure 1 Trigger points: side of head, neck, face and jaw

your earlobe and feel carefully along the length of each muscle for trigger points. When you come across an area that hurts, try to locate the nodule, then perform the deep stroking technique with your fingers, knuckle or a thumb. You may find that using a small rubber ball takes a little of the strain off your hands. Massage several times a day, until the trigger point no longer hurts at all when pressed.

Important note: Don't massage the area high under your chin where you can feel a pulse. There is a small possibility of loosening plaque into the artery here, and this can cause a stroke.

Prolonged back-tilting of the head – when painting a ceiling, for example – can cause contraction of the sternocleidomastoid and the formation of trigger points, as can keeping the head turned to one side. Trigger points can also be caused by curvature of the spine, a chronic cough, chronic hyperventilation (chest-breathing), emotional distress and habitual muscle tension. Further stress to the sternocleidomastoids can be prevented by taking heed of the following:

- Don't sleep on your stomach.
- Don't read on your stomach.
- Don't sit with your head turned to one side.
- Don't hold the telephone with your ear to your shoulder.
- Practise a deep-breathing and relaxation technique (as discussed in Chapter 5).
- Aim to correct your posture (see Chapter 2).

The trapezius

This great muscle structure is located across the shoulders and down the upper back. It attaches to the spine, collarbone, shoulder blades and base of the skull and helps to support the head and take the weight of the shoulders (Figure 2, 2). The trapezius is a major source of headaches and neck pain, for trigger points here can be wrongly diagnosed as migraines, neuralgia, bursitis of the shoulder, spinal disc compression and spinal stenosis.

The trapezius can be strained and trigger points can form when the head droops forward and the shoulders are rounded, as in a person with poor posture. In addition, tense people who carry their shoulders higher than normal will be at risk of developing trigger points. It can be seen, then, that someone in a desk job who rounds his shoulders and allows his head to droop forward may have problems, as may someone whose work dictates that his shoulders are kept raised. Women with heavy breasts are prone to developing trigger points in this muscle, as well. My best advice here is to improve your posture (see Chapter 2) and to take regular breaks from your work where you stretch your muscles. Women with heavy breasts should find that in addition to buying good, well-fitting bras with wide shoulder straps, improved posture can make a great deal of difference.

There are four possible locations for trigger points in the trapezius:

Location 1

Most people have a single trigger point in this location, and it can cause a lot of grief. It can be found by taking a pinch of the thin roll of flesh in the angle where the shoulder and neck join – not the bank of muscle at the top of the shoulder. A trigger point in the taut band here is the principal cause of temple headaches, usually self-

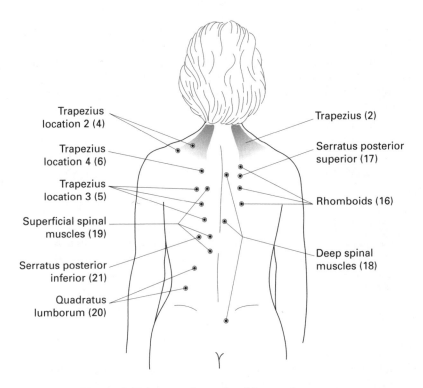

Trapezius location 2 (4)

Trapezius location 4 (6)

Trapezius location 3 (5)

Superficial spinal muscles (19)

Serratus posterior inferior (21)

Quadratus lumborum (20)

Trapezius (2)

Serratus posterior superior (17)

Rhomboids (16)

Deep spinal muscles (18)

Figure 2 Trigger points: shoulders and upper, middle and lower back

diagnosed as a tension headache. It can also refer pain behind the eye, into the jaw, down the side of the neck behind the ear, and occasionally in the back of the head (Figure 1, 3). Trigger points in this location can give rise to satellite trigger points in the muscles in the temple and jaw, causing jaw pain and pain in the gums.

Rolling the cord-like strand of muscle in the angle of your neck tightly between your fingers and thumb may reproduce a temple headache that will confirm it as the cause. Now perform the deep stroking technique. To save your hands, you may be able to position yourself so that you can use a ball against a wall. If this is too awkward, a massage tool be used, though be sure always to place a layer of cloth between the tool and your skin.

Location 2

The bank of muscle on top of the shoulder is a prime location for more trigger points. They can be present in pairs an inch or two apart, or be present singly (Figure 2, 4). They are often deeply embedded and are a primary cause of pain at the base of the skull, felt either as a headache or sore neck. Satellite trigger points can develop in the muscles at the back of the neck, causing further pain in the neck.

Most people will need to use a massage tool to work on trigger points in this location – a massage tool or a hard rubber ball is ideal. Remember to place a layer of cloth between the massage tool and your skin.

Location 3

Trigger points in this location can be found along the outer section of the lower trapezius, about halfway up the shoulder blade (Figure 2, 5). Like trigger points in location 2, they send pain to the base of the skull. Pain can also arise around the trigger point itself, and can cause a stiff neck and a burning pain in the mid-back. Satellite trigger points can arise in the same locality as original trigger points.

Moving a ball between your back and the wall is great for trigger points in this region. The ball will move either up and down or from left to right. Use whichever movement is easier, and which seems to offer the most relief. Go steadily, though, as it is possible to put on too much pressure with this action. Alternatively, a massage tool can be used.

Location 4

Trigger points in this location can be found in the broad inner part of the trapezius, between the shoulder blade and spine (Figure 2, 6). They cause a burning pain nearby, alongside the spine, and can be mistakenly diagnosed as spinal-disc compression, spinal stenosis, neuralgia or bursitis of the shoulder. Goose bumps on the back of the upper arm and thighs are a surprising result of trigger points in this location.

Although you may be able to reach any trigger points here with your hands, it is safer and less tiring to use a ball against a wall, or a massage tool.

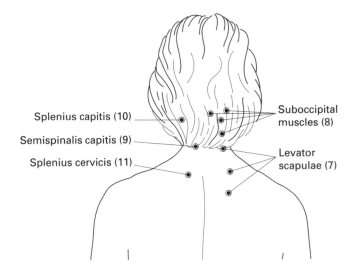

Splenius capitis (10)

Semispinalis capitis (9)

Splenius cervicis (11)

Suboccipital muscles (8)

Levator scapulae (7)

Figure 3 Trigger points: back of head and neck

Levator scapulae

It is common to have pain in the levator scapulae muscle, for it has the job of raising the shoulder blade. The upper section of each levator scapulae attaches to the top four neck vertebrae and the lower section connects to the upper angle of the corresponding shoulder blade (Figure 3, 7). Trigger points in the levator scapulae give rise to stiffness and pain in the angle of the neck, and they can make it impossible to turn your head to the side. Less common referred pain sites are along the inner edge of the shoulder blade and the back of the shoulder.

Trigger points in this muscle are difficult to reach, as they tend to be buried beneath the trapezius. However, you may be able to locate the lower part of the muscle, where it attaches to the upper angle of the shoulder blade. The central trigger point generally causes the most pain, but you'll need to apply strong pressure to locate it and then work it. The lower trigger point can be massaged by a massage tool or a ball against a wall, whereas the top trigger point is probably best worked by a supported thumb.

Tension from postural problems is a major cause of trigger points in the levator scapulae. Taking on board the following pointers should ensure that once trigger points in this muscle are cleared, they do not reappear:

- Don't lie on your side without a pillow to support your head.
- Don't hold the phone between your ear and your shoulder.
- Don't let your head droop when you're walking.
- When you must carry something on one shoulder – a shoulder bag, for instance – try not to tense the muscles of that shoulder.
- Don't use armrests that are too high or too low.
- If your shoulders always feel tense, try following the relaxation exercise in Chapter 5, on a daily basis.

Suboccipitals

There is a complex web of small muscles at the back of the neck which support the head and allow it to move. The suboccipitals are the most deeply buried of them all, located as they are at the very base of the skull. They are made up of four small muscles on each side, connecting the top two vertebrae to the skull and to each other (Figure 3, 8). They help to maintain the vertebral column in the erect posture, and serve to bend the trunk backward when it is required to counterbalance the influence of any weight at the front of the body, such as occurs in pregnancy.

Trigger points in the suboccipital muscles can cause pain in the head, in the forehead and back of the head. The pain is all on one side, which is typical of a migraine. If you suffer from migraines, you would do well to treat the trigger points in these particular muscles. Another cause of trigger points in the suboccipitals is neck stiffness and prevention of the tilting and nodding movements. Trigger points in the lowest of the suboccipitals can cause a stabbing pain in the side of the neck when it won't turn any further.

Although the suboccipitals are situated beneath other muscles, all the muscles here are relatively thin, so the suboccipitals can be easily reached. As it is important that you don't allow your head to fall forward during massage – this would cause the suboccipitals to contract – it is best to work on these muscles while you are lying on your back. Using alternate hands, the tool hand supported by the heel of the opposite hand, let your head fall back against your hands and carry out the massage with either your fingers or a small rubber ball.

To massage these muscles while you are in a standing position, you could use a massage tool, or a tennis ball held in the palm of your hand, the other hand placed at your chin to support your head.

Ensure that trigger points in the suboccipitals stay away by avoiding repeatedly turning your head or twisting around. Emotional tension can cause prolonged contraction of these muscles. Tackle this problem by perhaps seeing a counsellor or performing a daily relaxation routine, as described in Chapter 5.

Semispinalis capitis

These muscles connect the upper back and lower neck vertebrae to the base of the skull, allowing the extension of the head. Trigger points just below the back of the neck can refer pain to the back of the head (Figure 3, 9). Trigger points in the higher regions can send pain in a semicircle around the head, above the eyes and ears. As a result of trigger points in this muscle, there can be pressure on the occipital nerve that can cause numbness, tingling and a burning pain in the scalp at the back of the head.

Massage trigger points in this muscle with a ball or a supported hand.

Splenius capitis

There are two groups of splenius muscles – the splenius capitis and the splenius cervicis. The splenius capitis is made up of two bands of muscle that connect the neck vertebrae to the back of the skull (Figure 3, 10). They allow the extension and rotation of the head and neck. Trigger points in the splenius capitis send pain to the top of the head and are a prime cause of headache. They can be massaged by use of a supported hand.

Splenius cervicis

This pair of muscles connects the neck vertebrae to those of the upper back (Figure 3, 11). They allow for the extension and rotation of the upper back. A trigger point in the higher regions of the muscles can refer pain to the base of the skull, through the head to the back of the eye, causing blurred vision and symptoms typical of a migraine headache. Trigger points in the lower regions of these

27

muscles can create pain in the angle of the neck. Upper and lower splenius cervicis trigger points can cause the feeling of numbness or pressure in the back of the head.

Massage these muscles with a massage tool, or a ball against a wall.

Multifidi and rotatores

The deepest of the neck muscles, the multifidi and rotatores are numerous and tiny and run from vertebra to vertebra. They control the finer, more precise movements of the neck and head. Trigger points in these muscles can create severe pain on the spot and feel as though the spine itself is hurting. Referred pain can be experienced at the inner edge of the shoulder blade and the top of the shoulder. Satellite trigger points can occur in other multifidi and rotatores.

Extreme tension in the multifidi and rotatores is capable of partially dislocating a disc, as a result of which the vertebra is pulled to one side. Fortunately, deactivation of the trigger points can cause the vertebra to slip back into position.

Trigger points in these muscles can occur at any level and should be massaged with supported fingers. Alternatively, you could lie on a bed or the floor and allow a ball to do the work, gently moving your head from side to side.

Face and jaw pain

The majority of pain in the face and jaw comes from trigger points in the masseter muscle (see below), along with trigger points in the trapezius and sternocleidomastoid muscles (see the previous section). Trigger points in the smaller muscles of the face generally exist as satellites, and are likely to subside when trigger points in the larger muscles are cleared.

The masseter

The masseter (Figure 1, 13) is one of the most powerful muscles for its size in the body – 'masseter' coming from the Greek word for 'to chew'. The muscle originates in the lateral part of the cheekbone and inserts in the angle of the mandible (lower jaw). Its function is to raise the jaw, clench the teeth and masticate food.

Trigger points in the higher regions of the masseter, in front of the ear, can refer pain to the temperomandibular – the ball-and-socket joint that allows the lower jaw to open, close and move sideways on chewing and speaking. Contraction from trigger points in this muscle can be so great that it impedes the opening and closing of the jaw. It can even cause tightness in the vocal mechanisms. Other results of trigger points here are pain and sensitivity in the teeth, and pain under the eyes, over the eyebrows, in the ear and in the area of the sinuses.

Trigger points in the masseter can be massaged with supported fingers. However, most success is gained by placing the thumb inside the mouth and working the rubbery muscle between it and your fingers. Your thumb should be able to feel the rim of the sharp-edged bone called the *coronoid process*. Massaging the tender nodules can cause soreness for a couple of days. Try to endure it and carry on until there is no longer any pain.

To ensure that trigger points in the masseter don't recur, take on board the following pointers:

- Avoid chewing a lot of gum.
- Look after your teeth. Tooth decay, abcesses and excessive dental work can cause trigger points in this muscle.
- Breathe through your nose, not your mouth. Mouth-breathing causes tension in the jaw.
- Don't let your head droop. Poor head posture can make the masseter very tense.

Pterygoid muscles

Unfortunately, the wing-shaped pterygoid muscles (see 'Lateral pterygoid muscle' below, page 30) are obscured by the lower jawbone, which makes working on them difficult (Figure 1, 14).

Medial pterygoid muscle

Trigger points in the medial pterygoid muscle can cause pain in the ear and particularly in the temperomandibular joint, which worsens when you bite down. They can also send pain to the tongue, hard palate and back of the mouth, making it painful to swallow and to open the mouth wide.

Trigger points can be worked externally by pressing up with your thumb into the space behind the back of your lower jaw. Go carefully, however, as this spot can be very tender.

Lateral pterygoid muscle

Trigger points in this muscle are the prime cause of temperomandib-ular joint (TMJ) dysfunction. Persistent tension from trigger points in the lateral pterygoid muscle tends to pull the lower jaw forward and partially dislocate the joint, as a result of which cracking and clicking occurs on chewing. Trigger points here can also cause pain in the cheek that closely resembles sinus pain. They can even provoke sinus excretions, convincing the individual that he or she has sinusitis.

Trigger points in the lateral pterygoid can be massaged by placing the index finger inside the mouth and pushing it into the deep pocket behind the upper molars. After pressing back as far as you can, push inward and upward using tiny strokes.

Mouth-breathing or a lot of dental work, forcing you to hold your mouth open for a long period, can cause trigger points in the lateral pterygoid muscle.

Shoulder and upper-back pain

Trigger points in the muscles of the shoulder and upper back can cause a great deal of pain. The scalenes are included in this section, for although they are located in the neck, they cause a lot of referred pain in the shoulder and upper back.

Scalenes

The scalenes (Figure 1, 15) are a group of three or four small muscles of differing lengths at each side of the neck. They attach to some of the ribs and some of the vertebrae, and their main job is to lift the top two ribs on each side when you inhale. Trigger points in the scalenes are the cause of a great deal of pain, sending it into the chest, upper back, shoulder, arm and hand. Trigger points low in the middle and posterior (rearmost) scalenes are generally the cause of muscle-related chest pain, whereas trigger points high in the middle and anterior (frontmost) scalenes are generally the cause of pain in the upper arm and shoulder. The chest pain is sometimes mistaken for angina, and the upper arm and shoulder pain is frequently mistaken for tendonitis or bursitis.

Pain, swelling, weakness, numbness and tingling in the arm and hand are usually due to constriction of the scalenes, which can keep the first rib pressed up against the collar bone, squeezing blood vessels and the long thoracic nerve. This is called *thoracic outlet syndrome,* and is often misdiagnosed as carpal tunnel syndrome.

Access to the scalenes is difficult because they are overlaid by the sternocleidomastoid muscles. It is therefore necessary to familiarize yourself with the position of the sternocleidomastoids (see page 20). The anterior scalene lies between the sternocleidomastoid and the neck vertebrae and is almost completely hidden. The middle scalene lies behind the anterior scalene, around the side of the neck, with its lower section free of the sternocleidomastoid, and the posterior scalene lies almost horizontally behind the middle scalene in the triangular depression above the collarbone. Some people have a fourth scalene which lies vertically behind the anterior scalene.

To massage the anterior scalene, the worst culprit for pain, grip the sternocleidomastoid between your fingers and thumb. Let go with your thumb and, with your fingers, pull the entire sternocleidomastoid toward your windpipe, as far as you comfortably can. Now feel for trigger-point nodules on the firmer scalene from under your ear to down on your collarbone, where the most painful trigger points may lie. Massage them firmly against the vertebral column. Six one-inch strokes are sufficient at first.

The middle scalene can be reached by placing your fingers a little further back from the position of the anterior scalene.

The posterior scalene can be located by pushing your middle finger under the front edge of the trapezius, close to where it connects to the collarbone. Press downwards, then drag your finger toward your throat, parallel to the collarbone. You should feel the upper surface of your first rib as you search for and massage any trigger points here.

Trigger points in the scalenes are often created by laboured breathing, and can easily arise in people who suffer from asthma, bronchitis, pneumonia, emphysema and allergies. Laboured breathing after running or physical sport can also be a cause.

Once trigger points in the scalenes are deactivated, avoid the following to ensure they fail to return:

- Chest-breathing. Try to breathe deeply, drawing air into the diaphragm. (See Chapter 5 for instructions on deep breathing.)
- Playing a wind instrument.
- Carrying a heavy backpack.
- Working for long periods with your arms outstretched in front of you.
- Poor posture. Allowing your head to droop forwards puts the scalenes under a great deal of stress. (Follow my advice on the Alexander Technique in Chapter 2.)
- Emotional tension. The scalenes are perhaps the first casualties when there is habitual body tension. Listen to relaxation tapes, see a skilled counsellor if you have problems that are difficult to overcome, and follow my relaxation exercise, outlined in Chapter 5.

The rhomboids

The rhomboids (Figure 2, 16) are a pair of small muscles at each side of the upper back, running up diagonally to just below the base of the neck. They attach to several vertebrae and to the inner edge of the shoulder blade. The major rhomboid is lower and slightly separated from the minor rhomboid. These muscles raise the shoulder blade, hold it still, and move it toward the spine. Trigger points here send an aching pain along the edge of the shoulder blade. The scalenes are the most common cause of pain along the edge of the shoulder blades, so should be considered for trigger points first. A major indication that the rhomboids have trigger points is that your shoulder blades crack and crunch on movement.

Trigger points in the rhomboids can be massaged with either a ball against a wall, or a massage tool. Removing trigger points from the rhomboids will help you to hold back your shoulders and maintain good posture.

Once trigger points have disappeared, ensure they stay away by avoiding the following:

- Holding your shoulder blades stiffly pulled back for long periods.
- Activities that stress the rhomboids, such as rowing a boat or continuously throwing a ball.
- Any work dictating that your shoulders are kept up.
- Any trigger points in the pectoral muscles in the chest should also

be removed. If not, the muscle contraction they cause will pull the shoulder blade forward. In return, the rhomboids tighten in an effort to keep the shoulder blade in place. This tiring counter-activity is guaranteed to set up trigger points.

Serratus posterior superior

The muscles of the serratus posterior superior (Figure 2, 17) lie in the same direction as the rhomboids and also connect to the spine – however, instead of attaching to the shoulder blade they lie underneath it and attach to a few of the upper ribs. Trigger points here can cause a widely spread pattern of pain, overlapping the pain patterns of several other muscles. Referred pain includes a deep ache under the shoulder blade, in the back of the shoulder, the point of the elbow and the outer edge of the wrist and hand. In fact, pain in the little finger is characteristic of trigger points in the muscles of the serratus posterior superior.

To gain access to any trigger points in these muscles, move the shoulder blade aside by reaching the hand across to the other shoulder. Massage trigger points with a ball or massage tool.

Mid- and low-back pain

When you have back pain that persists for several months, it is only natural to suspect that something serious is going on – arthritis or disc damage, for example. In some cases of chronic back pain, the cause is chronic tissue disease or a mechanical problem, but in the majority of cases, the pain comes solely from trigger points in the muscles.

The deep spinal muscles

The muscles in this area of the spine are the *semispinalis*, *multifidi*, *rotatores* and *levator costae* (Figure 2, 18). They can be divided into two groups: the inner layers and the outer layers. Trigger points in these two layers often feel as though the spine itself is hurting. When trigger points arise in the muscles at the base of the spine, a sharp stabbing pain can result – one of the few examples of pain at the actual trigger-point site. The stabbing pain occurs because tension in the small muscles around the spine can pull one or more vertebrae out of line. Pain can occur adjacent to any of the vertebrae. Indeed, when there are several trigger points in the deep spinal muscles, movement can be severely restricted and disability can ensue. Chiropractic and osteopathy treatments are likely to reposition the vertebra(e) effectively, but until the trigger points are deactivated, the vertebra(e) are likely to be once more pulled out of line.

When there is extreme tension in the deep spinal muscles, the intervertebral discs can be damaged. Compression of the nerves can also occur, causing pain, numbness and tingling in the parts of the body they serve. Curvature of the spine (*scoliosis*) can result from extreme tension over a prolonged period. Indeed, experts believe that a proper understanding of trigger points by medical professionals could prevent the need for many spinal operations.

Referred pain from trigger points in the deep spinal muscles can be felt in the buttocks and even as far away as the abdomen. Furthermore, the tension resulting from such trigger points can cause a slight disarticulation of the sacroiliac, the fibrous joint that lies next to the spine and connects the sacrum (the triangular bone at the bottom of the spine) to the pelvis. Again, routine chiropractic and osteopathy treatment will fail to remedy the situation wholly when trigger points are the cause.

Many people are diagnosed with osteoarthritis when in fact trigger points are the culprits. The disc damage on X-rays can seem to verify the diagnosis and the person is prescribed painkillers as a matter of course, with no further investigation. However, back pain is often eliminated when trigger points are treated – even in the case of 'provable' arthritis. In a study, pain was found to be not always present in osteoarthritis – but where there were active trigger points, pain was always present.

Trigger points from the deep spinal muscles lie close to the spine, in the shallow dip between the spine and the bank of muscle on either side – the bank being the *superficial spinal muscles*. Using a small rubber ball against a wall is probably the best way to gain good access to these muscles, but go easily at first. Remember to make the strokes short and in one direction only. A massage tool may also be used.

The only time the deep spinal muscles are relaxed, besides when you are lying down, is when you are standing upright in a position that is posturally correct. Improving your posture, then, can ensure that trigger points do not reappear. Prolonged twisting and turning should also be avoided, as this causes stress to the deep spinal muscles.

The superficial spinal muscles

On each side of the spine, running over the deep spinal muscles, are three long muscles: the *iliocostalis*, the *spinalis* and the *longissimus* (Figure 2, 19). They run down between the shoulder blades to the bottom of the spine, starting fairly thinly in the upper back and getting gradually thicker. In the upper regions they attach to the ribs and in the lower regions they attach to the sacrum.

Trigger points in these muscles cause tightening throughout their length and a more diffuse type of pain than comes from trigger points in the deep spinal muscles. Trigger points in the longissimus and the spinalis are located within two inches of the spine and they refer their pain down to the low back and buttocks. Trigger points in the iliocostalis arise 3–4 inches from the spine and refer their pain upward and downward and slightly further to the side. One of the major causes of low back pain is a trigger point in the longissimus, on the lowest rib.

Trigger points in the iliocostalis can refer pain to the internal organs, where it can be mistaken for kidney stones, pleurisy and appendicitis. Pain can also be referred to the front of the body, where it can be mistaken for angina. Incorrect diagnoses are thought to include tumours, ligament tears, rib inflammation and disc problems.

The superficial spinals can be reached with a massage tool. However, massage is perhaps best conducted with the use of a tennis or high-bounce ball dangled over the shoulder and down the back in a stocking or sock. For trigger points in the lower regions of these muscles, try rocking the pelvis from side to side, putting more weight against the ball on alternate strokes. Massage can also be undertaken while you are lying on the floor, using your body weight against the ball.

When trigger points in this region are gone, protect the superficial spinal muscles by lifting more carefully, with your knees bent and your body straight and centred. Lifting while bending or leaning to one side is a sure way of setting up more trigger points in these muscles.

Quadratus lumborum

The quadratus lumborum (Figure 2, 20) is a pair of muscles that attach on each side to the lower rib, the lumbar vertebrae and the top of the pelvis. They control movement at the waist and largely support the upper body. As a result of trigger points in this muscle, coughing or sneezing can bring sharp stabs of severe pain, making it difficult to move. Other referred pain problems can be found in the hips, buttocks, groin, the base of the spine, the front of the thigh and around the sacroiliac joints. The muscle constriction from trigger points can hold one hip high and cause curvature of the spine, similar to scoliosis or a short leg.

Until you get used to the location of the quadratus lumborum, it can be best felt when you're lying on your back. Push your finger into the gap between your lowest ribs and hipbone and you will feel the solid wall of muscle that is the edge of the quadratus lumborum and the superficial spinal muscles. The quadratus lumborum is at the front of these muscles. Trigger points here can be treated by use of the supported thumb, a ball against a wall, or a massage tool.

Like the superficial spinal muscles, the quadratus lumborum can develop trigger points through incorrect posture when lifting – namely, twisting to one side to raise a heavy load. Emotional tension can cause trigger points here, too. Stop trigger points from reappearing by correcting your posture when lifting, and by seeking help for any emotional problems. See Chapter 5 for a relaxation exercise.

Serratus posterior inferior

The serratus posterior inferior muscles connect to the four lowest ribs and to four vertebrae in the lower back (Figure 2, 21). Their function is to help support the weight of the body during movement. Trigger points here can cause a localized ache that can be mistaken for kidney pain. Tightness in the muscle can cause restricted movement, particularly on bending and twisting.

The area around the ribs may contain several trigger points. They are best treated by using a massage tool or a ball against a wall.

When any trigger points have disappeared, avoid stretching, bending to one side or repeated twisting. Also, make sure that your mattress supports your entire body. Sagging mattresses cause a lot of problems for all the muscles of the back.

2

The Alexander Technique and posture

Trigger-point therapy is a direct, hands-on, treatment of pain. When accompanied by the Alexander Technique – a means of improving posture – the cause of the pain is often addressed, for poor postural habits are a major factor in the development of trigger points. If trigger points are deactivated but poor posture is not corrected, they will almost certainly spring back into life.

The Alexander Technique can be of benefit in treating a wide range of disorders, including backache, neck pain, migraine, headaches, muscle fatigue, depression, high blood pressure, circulatory disorders, asthma, speech defects, stomach ulcers, digestive problems and eating disorders. Even people with arthritis and rheumatic disease have shown great improvements after using the technique.

An innovative technique

Frederick Matthias Alexander (1869–1955) was a Shakespearean orator in Australia who excelled at solo shows. He carried his body and projected his voice as experts had taught him, but over time his vocal health began to seriously deteriorate. Unable to find a solution in the voice-training and medical approaches of the day, he resolved to help himself. Using an array of mirrors, he closely studied his posture and actions while reciting and was surprised to find that what he believed he was doing and what he was actually doing were entirely different. After further investigation, he developed a method that encourages all the body's processes to work more efficiently – the Alexander Technique.

Our sedentary lifestyles

The postural problems of human beings began quite recently, when we started to live less active lives. As hunter-gatherers in early times we were always on our toes, wary of danger and looking for food.

As farmers we were still very active, but the advent of the Industrial Revolution and machinery meant less physical activity. Today we lead sedentary lives. We have telephones, computers, cars, public transport, supermarkets, dishwashers, automatic washing machines and many other conveniences, and compared with the hunter-gatherer we use very little energy.

Stress

In today's modern world we use our minds far more than our bodies. We live in hectic environments with information to absorb and deadlines to meet. Whenever we face a stressful situation – such as a difficult work problem – the flow of adrenalin causes blood to be pumped into the muscles, and this may occur several times a day. The hunter-gatherers experienced stress in dangerous situations and they must have worried about where the next meal would come from, but the adrenalin was expended throughout the course of the next active few hours. Today we tend to exist with high levels of adrenalin in our bodies, adrenalin that is not naturally expended – and that creates chronic muscle tension. Some people find that the demands made on them regularly exceed their ability to cope. As a result, they feel stressed and overwhelmed. Health problems can ensue, such as headaches, tense shoulders, stiff neck, an aching back – often due to the formation of trigger points – and digestive problems, too.

Don't follow your instincts!

To his surprise, Alexander found he could not trust his instinct to determine whether his co-ordination, balance and overall posture were good, and he found it was the same with everyone else. They were all 'using' their bodies on the basis of a misleading instinct.

Test your own instincts

Close your eyes and try to place your feet side by side, parallel and even, on the floor, without touching each other. Now take a look. You are likely to find they are either pointing slightly away from each other or slightly towards each other. They may even not be exactly level. Yet they feel parallel and even. You can try this with your arms, as well. Close your eyes and stretch out your arms, trying hard to make your hands level. You will probably find, on opening your eyes, that your hands are not level at all. There may even be a surprising disparity between them.

We tend to think we can correct poor posture, movement and so on once we are told how to do it, and that then if we 'feel' we are doing it right, all is well. We now know that this is a delusion.

Bad postural habits

To break bad postural habits, it is a good idea to start as Alexander did and study your reflection in a full-length mirror. Most of us have come across our reflections in a mirror when out shopping and been surprised at our posture – and immediately corrected it. Maybe we have shortly afterwards seen ourselves in a second mirror, to find we have unconsciously reverted to that original bearing. Now is the time to hold that original – the one that was all wrong. Look searchingly at yourself in that full-length mirror and really absorb the way you are holding yourself.

Your shoulders may have felt as if they were even, but are you actually holding one higher than the other? Are they tense or drooping? Turning around slightly, you should be able to see whether you are holding your head high and straight, or low and forward, and whether your neck and the top of your back are drooping forward. Don't correct your posture just yet. Carry on with your inspection. It is only when you have absorbed the reality of your current body posture that you can start to work on correcting it.

Correcting posture

Changing bad postural habits can take a lot of effort – after all, they may have lasted since childhood. Emotional matters can play a part in how we carry ourselves, too. A shy girl who was perhaps bullied at school may have hung down her head and hidden behind her hair. A tall boy who was conscious of his height may have rounded his shoulders and constantly slouched to appear shorter. Teenagers with a growth spurt can do the same. Bad postural habits may just develop, however. Someone who twists to one side daily to read the newspaper spread out on the sofa can cause the spine to be out of alignment. It can be the same with people who must constantly turn to one side for their job – supermarket checkout assistants, for instance.

The basic premise of the Alexander Technique is that to keep the neck muscles from overwork, the head must balance lightly at the top of the spine. The relationship between the head and neck is of vital importance. How we manage that relationship has ramifications on the rest of the body. Indeed, whether the head and spine are compressed or free determines the excellence of the body's overall co-ordination.

Primary control

During Alexander's long period of experimentation, he learnt that the misuse of himself involved his whole body. He reasoned that to create optimum functioning of his body and its mechanisms he needed to lengthen his stature, and to do that he must allow his head to release forwards and up. When he was able to let his neck be free in this way, his back automatically lengthened and widened and his recitals were outstanding. He felt far more relaxed and before long his overall health was greatly improved. Alexander called the important relationship between the head and neck 'primary control'.

The string effect

Alexander observed that if the head and neck are properly aligned, the whole body follows into a natural, relaxed state. To find the correct postural position of your own head, imagine there is a string attached to the top of it and that it is gently pulling you upright. You have probably moved your head upwards slightly, your back will have straightened and you will have shifted yourself into a more upright position. Now repeat the process, but without actually moving at all. Because of the powerful links between mind and body, your mind will absorb the information and subtly start to control your body. Imagine the string is pulling you upwards in numerous situations, but again don't consciously act on it. Your subconscious will start to make corrections to your posture without your being aware.

Conscious projection

We know now that correct alignment of the head and neck allow good positioning of the whole body. But our instincts won't tell us what correct alignment is, so it has to be learnt. As well as imagining the string, try to recite specific instructions as often as you can. Alexander called these instructions 'conscious projection'. They should be as follows:

- 'Let the neck be free.'
- 'Let the head move forwards and up.'
- 'Allow the back to lengthen and widen.'

The above phrases are not things for you to do, but thoughts for you to think. They can be used like a mantra, repeated in spare moments – particularly when you are walking, sitting down, standing up or making other movements. The mind is a wonderful thing. After a while, you might think you have stopped listening to the mantra, but your mind will have absorbed the instructions and will be in the process of reprogramming itself.

'The means whereby'

We operate by what Alexander termed 'the means whereby'. In sitting down and standing up we have a means whereby we move and use our bodies. Alexander taught that 'the means whereby' is an important part of life. We all tend to concentrate on the end gain, such as the shopping we are about to do or the friend we are on our way to visit, and forget to enjoy the journey there. It's quite likely that our posture is very poor in our hurry to get where we are going – heads down, shoulders rounded, and bodies leaning forward. Alexander urged his pupils to concentrate on 'the means whereby' instead of the end gain, to relax naturally and move better. We are behaving like automatons when we fail to question 'the means whereby'. We move like human beings were meant to move when we examine 'the means whereby' and make a conscious decision to slow down and enjoy the journey.

The means whereby is not only relevant to the physical journey to a goal or end gain; it applies also to the way you carry out any task. This could include doing the ironing, writing a letter or loading a truck. As you get on with a task, ask yourself the following questions:

- How am I doing this task?
- How is my body positioned?
- Which muscles am I using?
- How do the different parts of my body feel in relation to the other parts?

Remember that simply being conscious of what you are doing will automatically allow you to relax and assume a better posture.

Inhibition

One of Alexander's most important discoveries was that if, just as he was about to do something, he let go of the thought of doing it, then his old habits failed to spring into action. He called this practice of letting go 'inhibition'. It allowed him to do something without being impeded by undue muscle stress and habits of poor posture. As a result, he was able to operate much better, whether when reciting or performing other activities.

The success of 'inhibition' lies not only in being able to stop just prior to an activity, it lies also in being able to decide upon the means whereby you want to tackle the activity. When an action is inhibited, you are letting yourself pause for breath and so become conscious of what you are doing. It gives you the opportunity to decide how the task can be done, what will happen if it's done and how you feel about doing it. The momentary pause will also allow you to decide whether the task should be done at all. The Alexander Technique is all about seeing what we do in a different light, then consciously finding a more efficient way of going about it.

When you have used the conscious projection of Alexander's 'Let the neck be free' and other mantras (see page 41) for a while, you should look closely at the means whereby you carry out your daily activities. Only when you think you are fully aware of how you go about things should you try to use inhibition.

It might help, at this stage, to think of your morning routine. You may already have observed how you wash in the shower, and later get dressed. Maybe not – after all, your manner of doing certain things will be so long-established that you may not even think about it. However, now is the time to analyse your actions. While in the shower, do you bend right over to wash your legs and feet, or do you balance on one leg – holding safely on to something, I hope – and hold up the other to wash it? When dressing, do you sit on the bed to pull on your trousers and socks or tights, or do you balance on one leg to pull them on? For now, just think about the way you undertake such actions. However, tomorrow morning, when in the shower, stop just prior to washing your legs and feet and ask yourself the 'means whereby' questions, and whether there's a better way of going about it than usual, a way that causes less stress to your body. As long as you are not in danger of slipping on the soap, you may want to lift up one leg at a time for washing. If this is not possible because of your pain, you could either ask your partner to wash your legs and feet for you, or you could sit in the bath and bring up your legs to wash them.

You could test inhibition while getting dressed, too. Just before dressing, stop and evaluate the situation to see if you can choose a way that is less taxing for your body. You know, it amazes me how we rigidly carry on in our routine, even when we have a pain problem that makes doing so very difficult. It was the same with me before my body virtually came to a full stop. Leaning right over to wash my legs and feet when my back was already hurting must have done me no good whatsoever; neither must balancing on one leg and stooping right down to pull on my tights. Such lack of care undoubtedly precipitated the worsening of my condition.

If you feel you now want to use inhibition properly, try to use it just prior to each action, remembering the way you were about to carry out the activity, then selecting a more efficient way. Performing an action in a way that is posturally correct becomes second nature surprisingly quickly.

A quick run-down of pointers so far

The Alexander Technique is an entirely new way of looking at postural problems, and as such can be difficult to absorb. Below is a breakdown of the main pointers we have covered so far. Don't try to rush from one instruction to another – you won't achieve anything. It may take a couple of weeks before you reach the stage where you are using inhibition.

43

Primary control. If the head and neck are in correct alignment – primary control – the remainder of the body will naturally follow on. Imagine there is a string gently pulling you upright, whether you are sitting or standing. Don't act on it. Imagining the string will be enough to make you gradually adopt a better body posture.

Conscious projection. Remember to repeat the following in spare moments: 'Let the neck be free,' 'Let the head move forwards and up,' 'Allow the back to lengthen and widen.' Don't physically do anything while you are repeating your mantra. Better posture will come from just saying these phrases to yourself, whether out loud or in your imagination. Their aim, rather than correcting your posture at that moment in time, is to reprogramme your mind.

The means whereby. Concentrate on the way you perform different tasks rather than on the end result. Focus on how your body is positioned, which muscles you are using and how the different parts of your body feel in relation to each other.

Inhibition. Just as you are about to carry out an action or task, stop and think, pause for breath. Now ask yourself what you will achieve by doing this task, whether it is suited to your capabilities and whether you really want to continue. If your decision is to go ahead, consciously choose the best way of going about it.

Stimuli

To get the most from the Alexander Technique, you should use inhibition in different situations, including at times of emotional upset. For example, a criticism may make you burst into tears, fly out of the room or shout back at the person. Inhibiting your immediate response will prevent that extreme reaction; it allows you to select a calmer response that causes you less stress. It can even enable you to see that the criticism was perhaps meant as a sincere, if clumsy, effort to help you.

The definition of 'stimulus' is a thing or event that evokes a specific reaction. A ringing telephone is a good example – the ringing being the stimulus for you to jump up and answer it, whatever you are doing. However, inhibiting your immediate response to the ringing allows you to determine whether what you are doing is actually more important. You can always ring the person back at a more convenient time.

Some stimuli trigger habits that are thoroughly entrenched. It is then difficult to inhibit that immediate response. A police siren or the wail of a fire engine or ambulance will immediately turn heads. We know it's nothing to do with us, yet we react all the same. 'Rubber-necking' as we drive past a traffic accident can cause not only a traffic jam, but also a further accident. Inhibiting that dangerous sideways glance can ensure that we reach our destination on time. It can also save our lives, and that of others.

The startle response

It might seem odd to read that our bodies are briefly startled when we are in the process of sitting down – but it is true. Our reflexes have barely evolved since the time of the early human, and as we begin to sit we temporarily lose our balance, falling backwards for a fraction of a second. The body reacts as if it is falling over. It tenses and prepares itself for injury, causing the blood pressure and pulse rate to increase, the heartbeat to speed up, the digestive system to shut down and the arteries to constrict. It also triggers the release of adrenalin, which can build up and cause chronic stress. When the body doesn't fall over, tension is stored in the muscles and other problems can ensue.

The Alexander Technique is all about understanding how we react to numerous stimuli and effectively changing responses that are harmful. Sitting is one of the major causes of tension in the body, so it is important that the process is relearned.

Sitting down

Human beings were built to stand upright, lie down or squat. Early humans would squat to eat, work and relax, whereas today we generally sit in chairs. However, it appears that chairs are designed with only style and ease of manufacture in mind, for they are often angular and hard. Humans, on the other hand, are soft and rounded. Furthermore, our thighs are not in their most relaxed position when at right-angles to our backs.

Alexander found that most people tilt back their heads and stiffen and shorten their necks on sitting. This exerts pressure on the whole spine, causing a distortion of its normal tensile condition. It also means there is less space for the internal organs, the lungs are restricted and the limbs are affected.

Some of our internal sensors work by detecting the position of our feet on the floor; they then tell the brain which muscles are required to support us. When we are lying down, the brain switches off all the muscles as it knows they are not needed for a while. It is only since humans invented chairs that our brains have become confused. When we are seated we may have either one or two feet on the floor and our brains are not sure of which muscles should support us.

The action of sitting

Using an upright hard-backed chair, try sitting down a few times. Be aware of the position of your head and neck each time. Now place your fingertips on the back of your neck and sit down again. Does your neck move backwards? Can you feel your neck muscles tensing? Most people use their hands to help lower themselves into a chair, letting go and falling when their bottom is about an inch or so from the seat. The startle reflex is thus triggered, causing the head to move backwards, the blood pressure and pulse rate to rise, the heartbeat to speed up, the digestive system to shut down, the arteries to constrict and adrenalin to be released – and this causes tension in the muscles.

Try sitting again, with your fingertips still at the back of your neck. As you ensure that your neck does not move backwards, lower yourself very slowly, keeping your balance all the time and feeling that you can stop whenever you want. In this way, the startle response will not be triggered and there will be no tension as you sit. Now, with your arms held loosely in front of you, practise sitting in this way several times. If you can lower yourself in this way all the time, you will find you are able to relax more when you are seated.

If your pain problem prevents you from taking the strain in your legs, try to use only chairs with arms. Hold on to the arms until you are fully seated and don't at any time allow yourself to drop.

Sitting crossed-legged

When our legs are crossed, the signals to our brains are confused. The postural muscles down one side of the body are switched on, whereas they are switched off down the other. Moreover, the spine is curved slightly to one side. If you sit with your legs crossed for a few hours every day, you risk backache and all the other symptoms that result from poor posture.

Standing up

To prevent muscle stress, it is important to get out of a chair, out of bed and out of a car correctly.

Getting out of a chair

To get out of a chair, allow your body to fall forward slightly, enough so you can then propel yourself further forward and up. To rise from a sofa, slide your bottom to the edge, then propel yourself into a standing position.

Getting out of bed

Levering yourself up prior to getting out of bed creates muscle tension. It can also strain the collection of nerves that lie alongside muscle fibres. The correct way to get out of bed is to roll on to one side and use the arm above to push yourself up into a sitting position. As you are in the process of pushing yourself up, let your legs swing over the side of the bed and on to the floor.

Getting out of a car

After opening a car door, we tend to grip the edge of the windscreen or the steering wheel and haul ourselves out of our seat. But repeatedly levering in this way can cause the collection of nerves alongside the muscle fibres to stop working.

The correct way to get out of a car is to swivel in your seat slightly so that your legs are out. Move your bottom to the edge of the seat, then let your body fall forward a little so you can propel yourself further forward and up.

Standing

Most of us have a posture that sags to some extent, which means we're out of alignment. Chronic pain can result in further misalignment, for pain often causes the body to droop and sag. When my own pain was at its worst, my head hung forward, my shoulders were rounded and there was a deep arch in my spine. I was gently told about my poor posture by the people around me, so I tried hard at times to stand straight and tall. I was aware of my poor posture and was making efforts to correct it, but what I thought was better posture was all wrong, and again my body was out of alignment. Now I was tending to hollow the small of my back and stick my behind and shoulders too far back to overcompensate. This is the way most people stand when they are thinking about it. Perfect alignment is different again and needs to be relearned. It feels strange when you first start to stand in the right way, but gradually it becomes second nature and feels right.

Out of alignment?

To discover whether you are out of alignment, remove your shoes and any thick clothing and stand with your back to a wall with your feet 45 cm (18 ins) apart and your heels 5 cm (2 ins) from the wall. Now gently lean back against the wall. Ideally, your shoulder blades and bottom should touch the wall at the same time, which means you are well aligned. If your shoulders touch first, you are holding your pelvis too far forwards, and if your bottom touches first, you are holding your pelvis too far back. If one shoulder blade touches before the other, you may be slightly twisted to one side.

Standing with your back touching the wall can feel quite strange, as if you are leaning backwards. In fact, you are standing more upright than you probably have for a long time. As you lean back against the wall, is there is a big gap between your lower back and the wall? If so, this is another indication of incorrect alignment. Try bending your knees, sliding down the wall until the gap disappears. Stay like this for a while, your arms hanging loosely at your sides. Take note of how it feels to have all three reference points touching the wall and so correctly aligned.

This position may feel uncomfortable at first, but will get easier with practice. Perform this exercise on a regular basis – at least twice a day – to help correct your body's alignment.

Walking

When you are out walking, do you look down at your feet? Most people do, and this means that your head is drooped forwards, your shoulders rounded and your neck and back curved. It's not good enough, either, to stop looking at your feet, although this is definitely a starting point. If you try to be aware of everything around you, scanning with your eyes as you walk, you will find that your natural instincts make you step up the curb or avoid that pothole. Modern humans tend to walk in the same way for all their adult lives. Often we recognize a person we know by their distinctive walk – and they probably recognize us by our distinctive walk. The trouble is, our distinctive walks are rarely good for us.

Changing your walk

It takes subtle reprogramming to begin to walk with our bodies correctly aligned. Reprogramming can start with that imagined string attached to the top of our heads, gently pulling us up, supporting and holding. Remember not to overdo the pull of the string. Walking stiffly upstretched is as bad for us as having a walk that is saggy.

The best way to correct your posture when walking is to lean back against the wall again, your feet 45 cm (18 ins) apart and your heels 5 cm (2 ins) from the wall. Bend your knees until the gap between your back and the wall closes up, then use conscious projection and inhibition. With conscious projection you will be saying, 'Let the neck be free', 'Let the head move forwards and up', and 'Allow the back to lengthen and widen.' With inhibition you will stop your normal walk. Now, without altering that posture, take a few steps forward from the wall. It's bound to feel strange. It's the link between walking like an ape and walking like a human. As you take a few more steps, let all the tension seep out of your muscles, let your arms hang loosely and make a comforting 'aahhhh' sound as you breathe out. Now slowly walk backwards to the wall. It is most likely that your bottom will touch first. Try it again and see which part of you touches. Your bottom? The aim is for your shoulders and bottom to touch the wall at the same time.

Practise standing with your back to a wall at least twice a day, sliding down the wall to gradually close that gap. Being careful to keep your back and hips in the same position, straighten your knees and walk away from the wall and around the room. Notice how quickly you revert to your old walk. Performed regularly, this exercise will gradually merge the strange new walk and your strange old walk. Watch out for the stage where you feel light and graceful. This is the walk you are aiming for!

49

Lying down

When we are lying down, we are choosing to be inactive. We are giving our bodies the chance to recover from the stresses and strains of previous hours. Being prostrate allows the back to lengthen, the shoulders to be released and broaden, and pressure to be removed from the joints. The pillow beneath your head should not be so high that your chin is resting on your chest, nor should it be so low that your head is forced back. Maximum relaxation can be achieved by lying on your back with your knees bent.

Writing

We usually crane the whole back and neck forwards in order to write. For people in desk jobs, writing like this all the time causes a great deal of stress on the muscles and joints. Try to inhibit this bad habit and instead take heed of the following pointers:

- Invest in a chair that supports your whole back.

- Move the chair as close to the desk or table as possible.

- Ensure that you are sitting upright, with your bottom pressed to the back of the chair.

- Tuck in your chin as you look down. This will reduce any strain on your neck.

- Bring your work closer to eye level. You may want to use a lap desk, a drafting table, or a secure box placed on top of your regular desk.

- Place work materials within easy reach.

- Tilt your head back every now and again to compensate for prolonged forward positioning.

- Take regular breaks. If you have a lot of paperwork to get through, keep getting up and walking around.

- Split the work into several short sessions. Try to alternate 'looking-down' tasks with duties where you can be more mobile.

Working at a computer

Using a keyboard or typewriter can stress the back, neck, shoulders, arms, wrists and hands. Follow the above recommendations and add in these:

- Use the computer's tilting feature to find the best position. When seated, the top line of the screen should be no higher than eye level. Too high a screen position will cause unnecessary neck strain.

- Ensure that the screen is directly opposite you. Looking to one side for prolonged periods can severely strain the neck muscles.

- If possible, adjust the height of your chair or work surface so your forearms are parallel with the floor and your wrists are straight. Sitting at a low work surface encourages poor posture.

- Invest in (or ask your employer for) a foot rest. This will reduce the pressure on your lower back.

- The mouse and other input devices should be positioned so that your arms and hands are in a relaxed and natural position.

- Position the keyboard directly in front of you. This makes it possible to type with your shoulders and arms relaxed.

- Position the mouse at the same level as the keyboard.

- When typing, keep your wrists in a straight and natural position.

- Keep your elbows in a relaxed position by your sides.

- Use the minimum force required to press down the keys.

- Purchase an ergonomic wrist rest for your keyboard. This should help to reduce (or prevent) tendon pain – similar to that of repetitive strain injury (RSI) – in your hands and wrists.

- Purchase (or ask your employer for) an ergonomic keyboard.

- Flex your hands and wrists every ten minutes.

- If required, use a wrist splint to minimize wrist mobility.

- If using a conventional mouse, move it with your whole arm rather than twisting the wrist.

- If possible, use a computer mouse containing a trackball. This will limit wrist movement.

- Use a 'moulded' mouse to support your hand and wrist.

- Take regular breaks. You will find that frequent, short breaks are far more beneficial than fewer, longer breaks.

- Stand and take a few minutes to stretch your muscles between breaks.

- Give yourself a time limit. When it is up, break off until later. (Should your pain levels begin to rise before your time is up, finish what you are doing immediately.)

Good posture in other activities

Taking on board the following pointers will improve your posture while you are performing all types of activities. If you also remember conscious projection and inhibition, any further strain can be prevented. As a result, you will start to function in a more natural, co-ordinated way.

Reaching up to perform a task

Performing an activity while reaching upwards – say, taking down crockery from a high shelf, replacing a light bulb, hanging curtains and so on – can put your back, shoulders and arms under great strain. It is best to:

- Stand on a small stool (one you know to be stable) so you don't have to stretch.

- Use a long-handled implement for inaccessible cleaning jobs.

- Take regular breaks to minimize strain.

- Store items in general use – such as groceries, pans, crockery and so on – in more accessible cupboards.

Washing up, preparing vegetables and so on

Leaning over kitchen work surfaces for prolonged periods can stress the neck and back. It is best to:

- Move as close to the work surface as possible to encourage proper posture.
- Stand tall, making sure to tilt your head down and tuck in your chin.
- Place a wooden box on the work surface to bring the work closer (maybe someone keen on DIY could make you one).
- Take regular breaks.
- Stop altogether as soon as you feel your pain levels begin to rise.

Carrying shopping etc.

Carrying heavy things such as shopping in your hands, your arms extended, exerts great strain on your shoulders, arms, and back. It is best to:

- Park your car as close as possible to the supermarket.
- Take someone with you so you can share the load.
- Limit the amount you carry at one time – two journeys carrying less is better than one journey carrying lots of bags or boxes.
- Carry packages close to your body, wrapping your arms around them. Carrying close to the body disperses the strain.
- Ensure that the load is balanced.
- Use a light wheeled shopping trolley rather than a full-size one, if available. Some of the big supermarkets offer the services of an assistant to take shopping to the car, so take advantage of this; one frozen-food retailer (Iceland) will do a home delivery if you shop in store. Alternatively, try internet or phone shopping and home-delivery services.

Lifting a bulky object up from the floor

Bending forward to lift something such as a full laundry basket can strain the whole back, the lower back being particularly vulnerable.

When lifting, you should be careful to ensure that your legs take the strain, rather than your back. The golden rule is, therefore, 'LNB' – which stands for 'legs, not back'. A reminder, too, that you must assess, first of all, whether or not you are really up to lifting. If you choose to go ahead, it is best to:

• Plant your feet about 30 cm (12 ins) or so apart. A wide base helps to maintain correct alignment.

• Keeping your back straight, bend your knees until you are resting on your haunches, then place your arms around the object.

• Push upwards with your legs to raise the object from the ground.

• If possible, break the load into smaller portions. Where laundry is concerned, it is safer to lift a few items at a time, carrying them close to your body (perhaps over your arm if the items are dry) to the washing machine, tumble drier or clothes airer.

Carrying a bulky object

Carrying can cause stress to the hands, wrists, arms, shoulders, neck and back. It is best to:

• Keep the object close to your body as you walk. Ensure that your grip on it is firm.

• Maintain an upright posture, again ensuring that your legs – not your back – take the strain (LNB).

• Rest the object on an available surface – a table or work surface – to give your muscles a break during the carrying time.

Setting down a bulky object

Placing a bulky object on the floor stresses the lower back in particular. It is best to:

• Plant your feet about 30 cm (12 ins) apart.

• Keeping your back straight, bend your knees, letting your legs take the strain as you lower the object to the floor (LNB once more).

• If transporting laundry, for example, from the kitchen to the outside washing line, setting the basket on a nearby patio table, garden bench or a broad-topped wall will save you the strain of lowering it to the ground.

Picking something light up from the floor

Most people tend to arch right over to pick a piece of fluff, for example, off the carpet. This can put enormous strain on the back – the lower back in particular. It is best to:

- Keep your back straight, bending your knees until you are able to reach the object.
- Use your thigh muscles to propel you upright again (LNB).
- If your leg muscles are too weak/painful to do the above, use a long-handled 'grabber'.

Placing a casserole in an oven

Bending forward at the waist whilst carrying with your arms outstretched puts a great deal of stress on your back. Holding something heavy away from your body increases that strain. It also stresses the tissues of the hands, wrists arms, shoulders and neck. If your oven is below worktop level, it is best to:

- Stand close to the oven, holding the casserole dish in both hands.
- Keeping the dish close to your body, drop down on to your haunches and slip the dish into the oven (LNB).
- Push yourself upright again with your thigh muscles. (Simply reverse the procedure to remove the casserole from the oven.)

Putting laundry into the washing machine

Bending to push clothes into the washing machine can stress your back and shoulders. It is best to:

- Lower yourself into a kneeling position, keeping your back straight.
- Push in only a small amount of washing at a time. Several repetitions are better than trying to thrust in a great bundle at once. (Reverse the procedure to remove the washing.)

55

Lying in bed all night

Lying down for long periods can make you feel stiff and sore. In particular, lying on your back puts a lot of pressure on your back and hips. It is best to:

• Place a pillow beneath your knees to take the strain off your lower back.

• Use no more than one small pillow to support your head and neck; moulded cervical pillows keep the head correctly aligned during sleep.

• Turn on to your side to relieve the pressure on your back and place a pillow between your knees to take the strain off your hips.

• Don't sleep on your stomach.

• Use a reasonably firm mattress. Mattresses that sag will contribute negatively to your problems.

Driving a car

Driving can stress virtually every muscle in the body. It is best to:

• Adjust the seat so it is near the steering column.

• Make sure the back of the seat is adjusted correctly; it should be neither too upright, nor reclined too far.

• Don't slouch or allow your head to droop forwards.

• Use a lumbar support (a cushion in the small of your back will do.)

• Make sure your car has a headrest. In the unlucky event of a collision, the headrest can minimize the severity of whiplash injury.

• Use your wing mirrors when reversing rather than turn around unnecessarily.

• When changing your car, go for power steering, if possible.

• When buying a new car, choose one with an automatic gearbox; this will eliminate the need constantly to depress the clutch and shift the gear lever.

- Electric windows, wing-mirrors, sunroof and so on are easier to manage than their manually controlled counterparts.

- Make regular breaks in a long journey to walk around and stretch your muscles.

- Share the driving with someone else.

Being taught the technique

It is not impossible to learn and practise the Alexander Technique on your own. After all, Alexander himself knew more about the technique than anyone else, and he was entirely self-taught. There are several books on how to self-teach.

Whether you can effectively practise the technique by yourself will depend largely on how much available time you have, how much you trust the technique and whether you have sufficient motivation to work on your own. The Alexander Technique is a complex system with concepts that are likely to be new to you – there is therefore little doubt that you will get far more out of being taught by a trained Alexander teacher than you ever could from following instructions in a book.

Is it safe?

Teachers of the Alexander Technique use their hands to guide the body, but they do so very gently, in a non-invasive way and using the minimum of pressure. It would be unlikely to cause any damage. However, if there is any concern about a medical problem, then a teacher may refer you to a doctor, particularly if a doctor has not yet been consulted.

Because the teacher works with you very closely, it is important that you feel at ease with him or her. If you don't feel at ease, find another teacher.

A typical lesson

During your first lesson, a case history will be taken; you will be asked about your daily activities and any sports or hobbies you indulge in, then the teacher will enquire whether you have any areas of concern.

As the lesson progresses, you will be taught the following:

- how the body operates
- how to use conscious projection
- how to sit, stand up, walk and lie down
- how to use inhibition in physical and emotional situations.

Pupils who master the dynamics of the relationship between the head, neck and back report more energy, increased freedom of movement, greater ability to cope with tasks and a better feeling about their bodies. In addition, the Alexander Technique can release long-held body tension, ease depression and anxiety and increase the ability to cope with problems. People with chronic health problems can make great improvements, too.

Finding a teacher

Look for an Alexander teacher with a certificate of membership from the Society of Teachers of the Alexander Technique (STAT) – these teachers will have the initials MSTAT after their name. Alexander teachers undergo a three-year, full-time training course that covers anatomy, physiology, the mind–body relationship and the significance of certain medical conditions to the technique. They will also have studied in detail the books written by Alexander and other relevant authors.

There are now Alexander Technique classes in most towns and cities, where a number of people are taught at the same time. The basic concepts can be put over very well in a class, and there is a certain amount of time given to each individual. However, most can obviously be gained from one-to-one instruction. Private Alexander teachers will come to your home, where you may feel more relaxed. Look in your local *Yellow Pages* directory or college prospectus for information about classes. Private teachers can also be found in the *Yellow Pages* directory. Best of all, get a personal recommendation, if you can.

3
Exercise

If you are in pain, exercise may be the last thing you want to think about. However, regular exercise can combat pain in a variety of ways. It prompts the release of endorphins, the 'feel-good' chemicals that can block pain signals from reaching the brain, and can also reduce anxiety and depression, conditions that can arise as a result of chronic pain. Regular exercise also improves sleep and provides you with more energy to cope with pain.

If you are using trigger-point therapy and the Alexander Technique, you may already be noticing improvements. However, if you have been inactive for a long period, your body will have become out of condition. Exercise of some kind is the only real way out of this state of affairs, I'm afraid. It may be different for those who have localized pain, for this has perhaps not impacted on your general fitness. In this instance, specific exercises can be used to strengthen the muscles around the sore area. For example, building up your arm muscles with strength training can provide a natural brace for an arthritic elbow.

When you first undertake exercise after a long spell of inactivity, the pain is likely to increase. This is because your muscles are tight and out of condition. Unfortunately, the only way to stretch and strengthen the muscles is to exercise them.

An individually tailored regime

An exercise regime should be tailored to your current condition. This will limit the chance of injury. The routine you devise should depend largely upon which exercises you are most able to do without too much pain, as well as upon which you most enjoy. If you are keen to strengthen a particular area in order to support a painful joint, choose the exercises that will build up the muscles around the joint.

As you read through the exercise possibilities, mark the ones you think you may be able to do. If only 'warm-ups' are within your scope at the outset, remember that you should be able to expand your routine as your muscles gain in flexibility and strength.

Take care not to overdo it

After warming up, perform one or two of the easier stretching exercises. If your pain levels are a good deal higher than normal the following day, either you did not allow sufficient resting time for your body to recover, or your chosen exercises were over-ambitious. Allow your body a further two or three days to recover, then recommence your routine with more basic exercises, and make sure you rest enough afterwards. As you finish your routine, you should feel as if you could have done more. You should be able to achieve the harder exercises when your muscles are stronger.

You may decide to aim for thirty minutes of exercise a day. However, to be safe, exercise for only a few minutes at the outset. And don't be in a hurry to increase your routine. Our muscles and other soft tissues respond far better to a slow and steady build-up.

Warm-ups

It is important to warm up and mobilize the muscles and joints before embarking on aerobic and weight-bearing exercise. This will increase your body temperature and the flow of blood to the working areas, preparing the cardiovascular system for exertion. Warm-ups also help to prevent muscular soreness and injury. Never skip warm-ups in favour of more vigorous exercise.

Stand with your feet about 40 cm (15 ins) apart, and keep your body relaxed, your back straight, your bottom tucked in and your stomach flattened as you perform your routine. All exercises should be smooth and continuous with the teachings of the Alexander Technique in mind throughout.

If you don't have full movement in any joint, stretch it as far as you can without causing yourself discomfort. You should find that you gain more and more flexibility as you continue to repeat the exercise.

Shoulders: Letting your arms hang loose, slowly circle your shoulders in a backwards motion. Repeat ten times. Now slowly circle your shoulders forwards and repeat ten times.

Neck: Slowly turn your head to the left, then hold to a count of two. Return to the centre and repeat ten times. Now turn your head to the right then hold to a count of two before returning to the centre. Repeat ten times. Tucking in your chin a little, tilt your head down

EXERCISE

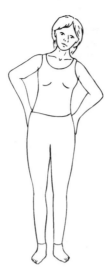

Figure 4 Warm-up exercises for the spine

and hold to a count of two before returning to the centre. Repeat ten times. Finally, tilt your head upwards and hold to a count of two before returning to the centre. Repeat ten times.

Spine (first set of warm-ups): Placing your hands on your hips to help support your lower back, slowly tilt your upper body to the left and hold to a count of two. Return to the centre, and repeat between two and ten times. Now tilt to the right and return to the centre. Repeat between two and ten times (see Figure 4).

Spine (second set of warm-ups): Keeping your lower back static, swing your arms and upper body to the left as far as they will comfortably go, then return to the centre. Repeat ten times. Now swing your arms and upper body to the right and return to the centre. Repeat ten times.

Hips and knees: Standing upright, lift your left knee upwards, as far as is comfortable. Hold to a count of two, then lower. Now raise your right knee and hold to a count of two. Repeat ten times (see Figure 5).

Ankles: With your supporting leg bent slightly, place your left toes

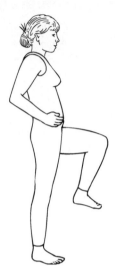

Figure 5 Warm-up exercises for the hips and knees

on the floor in front of you. Lift up your foot and then place your left heel on the floor. Repeat ten times. Now duplicate the exercise with the right foot (see Figures 6a and 6b).

Pulse-raising activities

Pulse-raising activities, another part of your warm-up routine, should build up gradually. Their purpose is to warm your muscles further in preparation for stretching. Marching on the spot for two to four minutes, starting slowly, then speeding up a little more is ideal.

Stretching exercises

Stretches prepare the muscles for the more challenging movements to follow, if you are up to them.

Calf (first set of stretching exercises): Stand with your arms outstretched and your palms against a wall. Keeping your left foot on the floor, bend your left knee. Press the heel of your right foot into the floor until you feel a gentle stretch in your leg muscles. Now change legs, alternating between the left and right leg. Repeat ten times (see Figure 7).

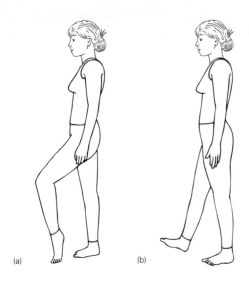

Figure 6 Warm-up exercises for the ankles

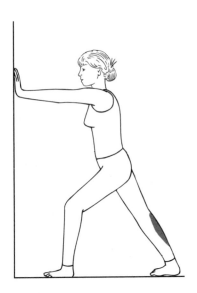

Figure 7 Stretching exercise for the calf

63

Calf (second set of stretching exercises): Standing with your feet slightly apart, raise both heels off the floor so that you are on your toes. Repeat ten times. As your calf muscles strengthen you should be able to stay on your toes for longer periods of time.

Front of thigh: Using a chair or the wall for support, stand with your left leg in front of your right, both knees bent, your right heel off the floor. Tuck in your bottom, and move your hip forwards until you feel a gentle stretch in the front of your right thigh. Now change legs. Repeat ten times (see Figure 8).

Back of thigh: Stand with your legs slightly bent and your left leg about 20 cm (8 ins) in front of your right leg. Keeping your back straight, place both hands on your hips and lean forward a little. Now straighten your left leg, tilting your bottom upwards until you feel a gentle stretch in the back of your left thigh. Now change legs. Repeat ten times (see Figure 9).

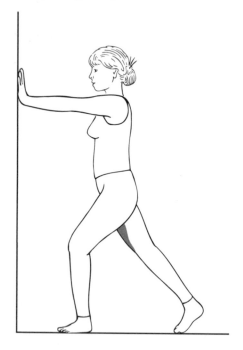

Figure 8 Stretching exercise for the front of the thigh

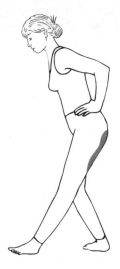

Figure 9 Stretching exercise for the back of the thigh

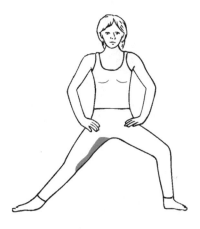

Figure 10 Stretching exercise for the groin

Groin: Spreading your legs slightly, your hips facing forward and your back straight, bend your left leg and move your right leg slowly sideways until you feel a gentle stretch in your groin. Gently move to the right, bending your right leg as you straighten the left (see Figure 10).

Chest: Keeping your back straight, your knees slightly bent and your pelvis tucked under, place your arms as far behind your lower back as you can. Now move your shoulders and elbows back until you feel a gentle stretch in your chest (see Figure 11).

Aerobic exercise

Aerobic exercise – an activity that makes you slightly out of breath – should come next. This type of exercise aids overall fitness and encourages weight loss. Try to choose an activity you will enjoy and want to continue.

Note that you should check with your doctor before embarking on regular aerobic activity.

Walking: This most convenient low-impact aerobic activity aids mobility, strength and stamina, and helps to protect against

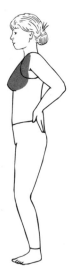

Figure 11 Stretching exercise for the chest

osteoporosis. You may find it easier to use a treadmill, reading a book or magazine at the same time or listening to a tape or CD player, the radio, or to audio (story) tapes. Aim to walk for 20 or 30 minutes at a time. A treadmill should never wholly replace outdoor walking.

Stepping: Start with a fairly small step (for example, a wide, hefty book, such as a catalogue or a telephone directory), or, if you wish, use a step machine or the bottom step of your staircase. Place first your left foot, then your right foot, on to the book or step. Now step backwards, first with your left foot, then with your right. Repeat for 2–10 minutes, then change feet, placing first your right foot on the step, then your left.

Trampoline jogging: Jogging on a small, circular trampoline can provide a good aerobic workout. If you can manage to get into a rhythm, the trampoline will do much of the work for you. Try to jog in this way for 20–30 minutes. Small, inexpensive trampolines are available from most exercise-equipment outlets.

Aqua-aerobics: Many people find aqua-aerobics, sometimes called 'aquacizes', both easy and enjoyable. Because the water supports your body as you exercise, it removes the shock factor, conditioning your muscles with the minimum of discomfort. The pressure of the water also causes the chest to expand, encouraging deeper breathing and increasing intake of oxygen. Rather than exercising alone in the swimming baths, most people prefer to join an aqua-aerobics class. The majority of public swimming baths run aqua-aerobic sessions, some of which are graded according to ability. As with all exercises, aqua-aerobics are only truly beneficial when performed on a regular basis. If you live a long way from the swimming baths, you will probably find yourself attending less and less, and then feel angry with yourself for eventually giving up. To minimize feelings of failure, be wary of undertaking activities that may be difficult to keep up.

Swimming: If you enjoy swimming, try to go to the baths once or twice a week and gradually build up the number of lengths you swim. Swimming exercises every muscle in the body in a way that causes them very little stress. However, as with aqua-aerobics or visiting a gym, you need to feel sure in yourself, before you start, that you will continue this type of exercise in the long term.

Cycling: Whether you use a stationary or ordinary bicycle, this form of activity provides an efficient cardiovascular workout. It is best to start by pedalling slowly and gradually building up momentum – and at first limit your sessions to two or three minutes, building up to 20 or 30 minutes, if possible.

Strength and endurance exercises

If you feel you have done enough at this point, run through the cool-down exercises and then congratulate yourself for doing something positive to help yourself. Perhaps when you feel fitter you can incorporate this section into your routine.

Thighs (first set of strength and endurance exercises): Lean back against a wall with your feet 30 cm (12 ins) away from the base of the wall. With your posture aligned, slowly squat down, keeping your heels on the ground. Now slowly straighten your legs again. Repeat between two and ten times.

Thighs (second set of strength and endurance exercises): Holding on to a sturdy chair and keeping your back 'tall', bend and then slowly straighten both legs, keeping your heels on the floor. Repeat the exercise between two and ten times. (See Figure 12.)

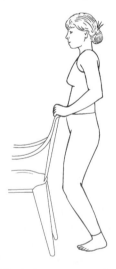

Figure 12 Exercise to strengthen the thigh

Upper back: Lie face down on the floor and, keeping your legs straight, gently raise your head and shoulders. Hold to a count of two, then lower them. Repeat between two and ten times. (See Figure 13.)

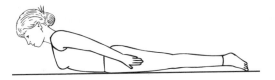

Figure 13 Exercise to strengthen the upper back

Lower back: Lie on your back and lift your right leg, pulling it towards your chest until you feel a gentle pull in your bottom and lower back. Repeat with the left leg. Now pull both legs up together. Repeat each exercise between two and ten times. (See Figure 14.)

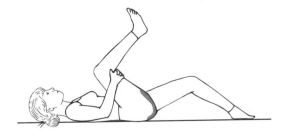

Figure 14 Exercise to strengthen the lower back

Abdomen: Lie on your back with your knees bent and your feet flat on the floor. Now raise your head and shoulders, reaching with your arms towards your knees. Remember to keep the middle of your back on the floor. (See Figure 15.)

Push-ups: Stand with your hands flat against a wall, your body straight. Carefully lower your body towards the wall, then slowly push away. Repeat two to ten times. (See Figures 16a and 16b.)

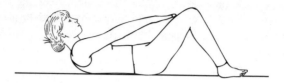

Figure 15 Exercise to strengthen the abdominal muscles

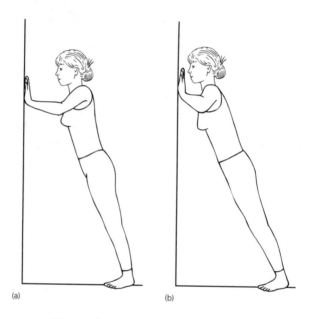

(a)   (b)

Figure 16 Push-ups against the wall

Using weights

Exercising with weights can form a useful part of your strength and endurance routine. You could use a bag of sugar, a tin of beans, or the Velcro weights that strap around the wrists or ankles. It shouldn't be necessary to use anything heavier.

Fasten the weights around your wrists or hold them firmly in each hand, then stand with your feet slightly apart. Now try the following:

- Keeping your left elbow close to your waist, slowly raise your left forearm so that it almost touches your shoulder. Lower the arm until it is at right-angles with your upper arm, then slowly raise it again. Ensure that the movements are slow and continuous. Repeat between two and ten times. Build up the repetitions in line with your level of fitness.
- Making sure that only your upper body moves, turn to the left, swinging both arms as you move. Repeat two or ten times. Now perform the same exercise and number of repetitions, swinging your body and arms to the right. Ensure the movements are slow and fluid. Build up the repetitions in line with your level of fitness.
- Bend your left arm so that your elbow is down and your forearm upright (in other words, so that your wrist is at your shoulder), then raise your arm upward until your elbow is straight. Bring it back down to the original position. Repeat once more, then do the same with your right arm. Repeat between two and ten times. Build up the repetitions in line with your level of fitness.

Finish your routine by cooling down, using the warm up exercises given above.

Exercise routine

Ideally, you should carry out your routine three or four times a week. Try to exercise before breakfast, if possible. The low levels of insulin in your body at that time allow access to body fat for conversion to energy. To boost your fitness levels further – especially if you are not able to perform a regular aerobic regime – try walking to work, walking to the shops, getting off the bus a stop or two earlier, and taking the stairs instead of the lift. Remember, most of all, that every little helps.

4
Nutrition

You may wonder how good nutrition could possibly be described as a pain-beating technique. Nutritionists are in no doubt, however, that eating the right foods helps to combat pain. The effect is rather less immediate than that of some other treatments – painkillers, for instance. However, painkillers give only temporary ease, whereas the benefits of good nutrition occur at a much deeper level and with far-reaching consequences of a very positive nature.

Changing the way you eat can change the way you feel. In the short term, it provides extra energy, lifts mild to moderate depression, reduces aching, and gives a sense of well-being. In the long term – especially when used in conjunction with trigger-point therapy, exercise and the Alexander Technique – it can keep you free from pain, inflammation, stiff joints and fatigue. It will also promote longevity and overall good health.

The diet that can best fight pain is primarily an organic, wholefood diet consisting largely of fruits and vegetables, nuts and seeds, fish, grains and oils. These foods are high in dietary fibre, which means they help to move food and waste products through the digestive tract before they have a chance to form toxic substances. It is thought that pain problems are far more likely to occur in people who consume little fibre.

Having read that these are the recommended foods, don't panic just yet! Absorb this chapter before you make your decision as to whether you want to change your diet. I have included a number of 'summing-up' pointers to make your transition to healthy eating as easy as possible.

Sins of the modern diet

Crop production today is loaded with chemicals. More are then added to allow foods to travel long distances; to help them to withstand a long shelf life, to keep them looking fresh and to enhance the flavour. However, foods that have been refined and processed in this way are depleted in nutrients and the chemical content is known to be harmful to health (Hall, 1981).

The following points outline current food habits:

We eat food that has been sprayed many times with chemical pesticides, herbicides and fungicides. These poisons kill essential soil microbes that would otherwise help plants to absorb nutrient-rich minerals such as zinc, copper, magnesium and manganese. These minerals are essential to good health.

We also eat food grown on land that has been artificially fertilized with nitrogen, potassium and phosphorus instead of manure or compost. Although artificial fertilizers stimulate plant growth, their use has greatly reduced the mineral content of the soil concerned. It also causes an imbalance in our hormone levels. Organically grown foods may be a little more expensive, but they are toxin-free and they do taste good.

Plant foods are then artificially ripened, stored and processed. Unfortunately, the refining and storage process robs food of the majority of its fibre and nutrients. Most of the precious B vitamins and vitamin E are lost in the processing and bleaching of wheat and flour, leaving it valueless and slightly poisonous to the body. Similarly, all other cereals, fruits and vegetables lose much of their nutrients and vitamin C during processing.

Finally, we eat the tasty parts of the food only, disposing of the rest. For example, wheat husks and wheatgerm – the most nutritious parts of the plant – are removed before the remaining cereal is processed into white flour. 'Whole' foods contain fibre and so aid the removal of waste materials from the bowel. They are vital to good bowel health.

Cutting out food additives

Cutting out additives such as food colourings, preservatives and flavourings (usually listed on the tin or packet as 'E numbers') should ensure that you consume fewer toxins. This can also go a long way toward rebalancing the body.

Unfortunately, the majority of the foods on our supermarket shelves have undergone some degree of chemical refinement or alteration. The additives that cause most harm are monosodium glutamate (MSG), artificial colourings, butylated hydroxyanisole (BHA), butylated hydroxytoluene (BHT), sorbate, sulphites and aspartame.

Contrary to popular belief, aspartame will not help you to lose weight. It is known to trigger a craving for carbohydrate and will cause an increase in weight. At a recent World Environment Conference, one doctor revealed that when he got people off aspartame, their average weight loss was 8.5 kg (19 lbs) per person. Aspartame is commonly found in foods described as 'low sugar', 'sugar free', or 'diet'. Equal and NutraSweet are brand names for this product.

Other foods to avoid

People with a pain problem should try to avoid acid-forming foods. Pain can cause the body tissues to be overly acidic, which encourages inflammation and increases the risk of inflammatory disease. Foods that raise acid levels are sugar and refined carbohydrates, alcohol, vinegar, coffee, meat and dairy products. Foods that increase alkalinity and therefore reduce acidity are all vegetables and foods with green leaves or a green skin.

This section gives the foods that should, ideally, be limited.

Reducing sugar and refined carbohydrates

Our diets are often high in sugar and refined carbohydrates (biscuits, cakes, pastries, etc.) – food that has little nutritional value and uses a great deal of energy in its digestion, absorption and elimination. Sugar and refined carbohydrates are acid-forming foods and should really be avoided.

Sugar consumption has been linked with many disorders, from diabetes to heart disease and cancer. You probably know that sugar converts into energy. What you may not know is that we can obtain all the sugars/energy we need from fruit and complex (unrefined) carbohydrates (grains, lentils, etc.), which convert into sugar in the body as nature intended.

Reducing salt

Salt is commonly used as a preservative and is added to most processed, pre-packaged foods; cornflakes, for example, are high in salt. As a result, people may be consuming more salt than they realize, especially when that used in cooking and at the table is taken into account. However, *whole foods* actually contain salt (sodium) and potassium in just the right balance for our bodies. Extra salt upsets this happy balance and can lead to a variety of problems. Try using herbs and spices for flavouring (in moderation). Sea salt contains more minerals than ordinary salt, but it is still salt – so use sparingly.

Reducing caffeine products

If too much caffeine is consumed – caffeine products include coffee, cocoa, cola drinks and chocolate – stress can occur to the liver and adrenal glands, and the body's ability to absorb vitamins and minerals can be seriously impaired. It can also cause enough metabolic irregularity to make it difficult to keep trigger points deactivated. So how much is too much? After a flurry of studies into the effects of caffeine, experts have now concluded that 300 mg daily of coffee, or 2–3 cups, is safe. This roughly equates to one can of cola drink, or 2–3 cups of cocoa, or one bar of chocolate.

A problem for many is finding an acceptable alternative to caffeine. Coffee, cocoa and cola drinks can be replaced by fruit and vegetable juices, or herbal teas; green tea is very good (see below), as is rooibosch (redbush) tea. They are both low in tannin and high in antioxidants. A variety of grain coffee substitutes may also be purchased from health-food shops. Since many decaffeinated products are processed with the use of chemicals, they are not a good choice.

Carob, similar to the cocoa bean, is a healthy, caffeine-free alternative to cocoa and chocolate. It contains less fat and is naturally sweet, unlike the cocoa bean, which is bitter and needs sweetening. Many people find carob bars an enjoyable replacement for chocolate bars and other confectionery. It is also available in powder form for use in baking and in drinks.

Reducing red meat and dairy produce

It is recommended that people with a pain problem cut down on saturated fats from dairy produce and red meat. These products are acid-forming and increase the potential for developing further inflammatory conditions.

White meat and fish – particularly oily fish such as herring, mackerel, sardines and tuna – are good sources of protein and oils, but a piece no larger than the palm of your hand should be eaten in a day. Try to ensure that any meat and fish you buy is organic – that is, from animals reared without the use of antibiotics, anabolic steroids, chemical pesticides and so on.

Dietary fats

Fats (fatty acids) are the most concentrated sources of energy in our diet, one gram of fat providing the body with nine calories of energy. However, as you may be aware, some fats are beneficial to health while other fats are capable of raising cholesterol levels and causing knock-on health problems.

Fats can be categorized as follows:

Saturated fat: Associated with the development of degenerative disease, including heart disease and even cancer, saturated fat comes mainly from animal sources and is generally solid at room temperature. Margarine was, for many years, believed to be a healthier choice than butter, but nutritionists have now revised their opinion. It seems that some of the fats in the margarine hydrogenation process are changed into trans-fatty acids, which the body metabolizes as if they were saturated fatty acids – the same as butter. Butter is a valuable source of oils and vitamin A, but should be used very sparingly. Margarine, on the other hand, is an artificial product containing many additives.

Unsaturated fat: Also called polyunsaturated or monounsaturated fat, unsaturated fat has a protective effect on the heart and other organs. Omega 3 and omega 6 oils occur naturally in oily fish (mackerel, herring, sardines, tuna, etc.), nuts and seeds, and is usually liquid at room temperature. Olive, rapeseed, safflower and sunflower oil are types of unsaturated fat.

Frying

It is important to note that the process of *frying* changes the molecular structure of foods, rendering them potentially damaging to the body. If you must fry something, it is best to use a small amount of extra-virgin olive oil and to cook at a low temperature. A healthier alternative is to sauté in a little water or tomato juice, or to grill, bake and steam. 'Stir-frying' is good, but cook the food in a little water, drizzling olive oil on afterwards.

It is important to remember never to reheat used oils, for this, too, can be harmful to the body. Store your oils in a sealed container in a cool, dark place to prevent rancidity.

Eggs

You are no doubt aware that eggs are high in cholesterol, which is a type of fat. However, they also contain lecithin, which is a superb biological detergent capable of breaking down fats so that they can be utilized by the body. Lecithin also prevents the accumulation of too many acid or alkaline substances in the blood and encourages the transportation of nutrients through the cell walls. Eggs should be soft-boiled or poached, as a hard yolk will bind the lecithin, rendering it useless as a fat-detergent.

Although it is recommended that you eat two or three eggs a week, those following this diet on a vegetarian basis should eat up to five eggs a week to obtain the necessary protein.

A 'whole-food' diet

Whole foods are simply those that have had nothing taken away (i.e. nutrients and fibre), and that have had nothing added (i.e. colourings, flavourings, preservatives, etc.). In short, they are foods in their most natural form. Whole foods that are organically produced – without the use of chemical fertilizers, pesticides and herbicides – are even better for us.

A rough outline of the foods recommended is as follows.

Fresh fruit and vegetables

As stated, arthritis and other inflammatory diseases are known to raise levels of acid in the body. Vegetables, however, provide a great alkaline leveller. As a rule of thumb, the greener the vegetable, the more it will help to reduce acidity and therefore inflammation and pain.

Grapes contain resveratrol, a plant-derived non-steroidal compound that works to block inflammation. So, snack on grapes or add them to salads (wash them first).

For many years, professional coaches have encouraged their athletes to eat pineapple to help heal sports injuries. Pineapple contains a key enzyme called bromelain, which works to reduce inflammation – a fact substantiated by a German study. Other studies have shown that eating pineapple can ease the pain and tissue-swelling of carpal tunnel syndrome.

People low in glutathione, a powerful antioxidant and detoxifying agent, are more likely to suffer from arthritis and joint inflammation than those with higher levels, according to research. Glutathione is present in broccoli, cabbage, asparagus, cauliflower, tomatoes and potatoes. Fruits with this agent include avocados, oranges, grapefruit, peaches and watermelon.

Try to buy locally grown, organic fruit and vegetables that are in season. They have the highest nutrient content and the greatest enzyme activity. Enzymes are to our body what spark plugs are to the car engine. Without its 'sparks', the body doesn't work properly. Organically grown fruit and vegetables may not look as perfect as those that are processed, but they *are* superior – processed foods are devitalized of their 'sparks'.

Eat your vegetables as raw as possible. Make a variety of salads and try to eat one every day. When you do cook vegetables, cook them in the minimum of unsalted (or lightly salted) water for the minimum of time. Lightly steaming or stir-frying are healthy alternatives. Scrub rather than peel.

Legumes (peas and beans)

In a study at the American Pain Society, researchers saw that a diet rich in soy quickly reduced pain and swelling in rats, and it is surmised that the same pain tolerance might be seen in humans who eat a lot of soy.

Soy foods have other great benefits: they are high in protein, dairy-free, low in saturated fat, an excellent meat substitute, and can be purchased as soya milk, tofu, tempeh and miso. Tofu, for example, is very versatile and can be used in both sweet and savoury dishes.

Butter beans, mung beans, chick peas, haricot beans, lentils, garden peas, kidney beans and split peas are, like the soya bean, rich in phytoestrogens and should be consumed as often as possible.

Seeds

Sunflower, sesame, hemp and pumpkin seeds contain a wonderful combination of nutrients, all necessary to start a new plant. They can be eaten as a snack, sprinkled on to salads and cereals, or used in baking. For more flavour they can be lightly roasted and coated with organic soy sauce. Cracked linseed is also highly nutritious, and useful for treating constipation. It can be used in baking and sprinkled on to breakfast cereals and porridge oats.

Nuts

All nuts contain vital nutrients, but almonds, cashews, Brazils and pecans offer the greatest array. Eat a wide assortment as snacks, with cereals and in baking.

Oils

In the 1970s, the diet of the Inuit people of Greenland was put under the microscope, for it was realized that these people were suffering far less from heart disease, arthritis, lupus, diabetes, psoriasis and even, in women, menstrual pain than their European counterparts. It was quickly seen that they consume a great deal of foods containing omega 3 oils. Fortunately, we don't need to eat whale and seal meat to obtain this important oil, for it also occurs in salmon, tuna, herring, mackerel, anchovies, sardines, sturgeon, whitefish and other oily fish.

Omega 6 oil is important too, and can be obtained from nuts, seeds, cereals and wholegrain bread. It is recommended that people with a pain problem eat oily fish at least three times a week and use cold-pressed oil daily for dressings, such as olive oil, rapeseed oil, canola oil, flaxseed oil, safflower oil and sunflower oil. Olive oil is best suited to cooking, as it suffers less damage from heat than other oils.

Grains

Wheat is our staple grain in the west; however, refined wheat flour means that the nutritious husks and germ have been removed including vitamins, minerals, protein and the fibre. Only carbohydrates, calories and a little protein remain.

Fortified flours have had some of their nutrients replaced. However, vitamin B6, vitamin E and folic acid are not put back. Also, of the nine minerals initially removed, only three – iron, calcium and phosphorus – are returned, but in forms that are not easily absorbed by the body. All in all, refined flours have little nutritional value.

Healthy flours include whole-wheat flour, spelt flour, quinoa flour, oat flour, maize flour, brown-rice flour, rye flour, barley flour and potato flour, all of which are high in nutrients. Buckwheat, although not actually a grain, also makes a delicious alternative, and, like millet and rice, is free of gluten, a common allergen. Because wheatgerm is high in the B vitamins that are so important to people with a pain problem, it is highly recommended. Granary bread, to which crushed wheat and rye grains have been added, makes a pleasant alternative. Remember that organically produced flours are best.

A word of warning. Please ensure that your 'wholemeal' loaf of bread really *is* wholemeal and not dyed white or a mix of flours. I'm afraid 'brown' tells you nothing. Bread mixes that are nutritious and easy to prepare can be purchased in health-food shops.

Aim to consume a variety of grains. Oats are highly recommended, as they help to stabilize blood-sugar levels.

The benefits of green tea

Green tea contains an important substance that inhibits inflammation. In fact, researchers believe that several cups of green tea daily can not only reduce inflammation and pain, but can also improve overall health.

A sample menu

To give you a better idea of the type of foods recommended, I have devised a seven-day sample menu. If the foods here are very different from your current diet, please don't be daunted. This menu is an ideal, something you might want to aim for over a period of time.

Drinks should include plenty of water, herbal teas, green tea and fresh fruit and vegetable juices. All fruit and vegetables should be organic, all bread wholemeal, and any pre-packaged foods should be free from additives.

'Cup' means a small teacup or American cup measure rather than a mug.

Day 1

Breakfast   Grilled sardines on two slices of wholemeal toast
Snack   Carob bar

Lunch	Bean and vegetable soup with two wholemeal rolls; pear
Snack	$\frac{1}{3}$ cup mixed dried fruit and nuts
Dinner	Home-made chicken curry with brown rice
Snack	Two slices wholemeal toast

Day 2

Breakfast	Grapefruit with a little muscovado sugar and two slices wholemeal toast
Snack	$\frac{1}{3}$ cup mixed sunflower seeds and almonds
Lunch	A salad of your choice, with low-fat mayonnaise and no cheese; apple
Snack	$\frac{1}{3}$ cup dried apricots
Dinner	Irish stew with a little beef and plenty of vegetables
Snack	Two oatcakes

Day 3

Breakfast	Porridge with cracked linseed, rice milk and a little muscovado
Snack	Orange
Lunch	Two grilled kippers with two slices of wholemeal bread
Snack	$\frac{1}{4}$ cup of mixed walnuts and pecan nuts
Dinner	Mixed vegetable casserole
Snack	Two Ryvita crackers with cottage cheese

Day 4

Breakfast	Organic raisin bran with chopped banana
Snack	Two rice cakes
Lunch	Mixed salad; baked apples
Snack	Pear
Dinner	Baked wild salmon with potatoes, broccoli and carrots
Snack	Two oat cakes

Day 5

Breakfast	Porridge with cracked linseed, raw honey and rice milk
Snack	Two kiwi fruit
Lunch	Two soft-poached eggs on two slices of wholemeal toast

Snack	$\frac{1}{3}$ cup pecan nuts
Dinner	Grilled chicken breast with potatoes, carrots and green beans
Snack	Apple

Day 6

Breakfast	Large wedge of cantaloupe melon
Snack	Two oatcakes
Lunch	Tuna salad; banana
Snack	$\frac{1}{3}$ cup dried apricots
Dinner	Falafel (similar to a veggie-burger and available from health-food shops) with beans and home-made oven chips; orange
Snack	Two farmhouse biscuits

Day 7

Breakfast	Fresh fruit salad
Snack	Two Ryvita crackers with cottage cheese
Lunch	Baked potato with baked beans; apple
Snack	$\frac{1}{3}$ cup mixed nuts
Dinner	Tuna salad with two wholemeal rolls
Snack	Orange

Making changes

Changing the habits of a lifetime takes a great deal of determination. We are used to choosing foods that satisfy our taste buds – they are often made tastier by the addition of chemical flavourings, fat, sugar, salt and so on – and may be loath to make drastic changes. So, alter your eating habits gradually, allowing yourself time to adjust to the new textures, appearance and flavours of different foods. And a word of warning about sudden dietary changes: nutritious, cleanly-grown foods may trigger the body into instant detoxification, causing headaches, lethargy and even diarrhoea. This shock to the system will be avoided if you take the following step-by-step approach to your new way of eating:

Change only one meal a day to healthy eating at first – it doesn't have to be a particular meal. You could have a healthy main meal one day and a healthy breakfast the next. Try to remember that it takes only 28 days of eating a food regularly for it to become a habit. Three or four weeks later you may be ready to introduce a second healthy meal per day.

The changeover will be easier if you cook double the amount of main meal required. You can then heat up the rest the next day. Don't freeze foods too often, as this can kill important nutrients.

When introducing the new diet, remember that it is necessary to eat a wide variety of foods to supply the vital building blocks of life.

Cut down on snack foods such as crisps, chocolate bars and biscuits. Gradually replace them with fresh fruit, dried fruit, nuts, seeds, carob bars, muesli bars, oatcakes and so on. If you drink a lot of carbonated beverages such as cola and lemonade, phase them out slowly and introduce green tea, fruit juices, soya milk and so on.

When eating out, select a restaurant with healthy choices on the menu. Don't be afraid to ask the chef to modify a dish – leaving out a cream sauce, for example.

If there are foods in the sample diet you just know you wouldn't eat on a regular basis, cut them out of your mind. A long-term diet will only work if it is practical, sustainable and compatible with your lifestyle. If you feel it would be too difficult to change over to healthy eating on your own, you may want to ask your doctor for a referral to a dietician for help. Alternatively, there are many excellent nutritionists who can offer skilled guidance, for a fee.

Nutritional supplements

Studies into the most common diseases have shown they create certain vitamin and mineral deficiencies. To ensure that you get a balance of vitamins, minerals and other essential nutrients, you may wish to take nutritional supplements.

Supplements should be taken before meals to ensure maximum absorption. Look for supplements without added colourings, flavourings, preservatives, hydrogenated fats, gelatine and sugar – and check the strength. Sadly, some brands of supplements contain only small amounts of the active ingredients. A good company will have a qualified nutritionist available to answer telephone queries and will train retailers to know about their products. Of course, they may still be biased towards their own products!

Magnesium and malic acid

Supplements of magnesium and malic acid (or magnesium malate) have been shown to reduce pain and fatigue markedly. Magnesium plays a vital role in the operation of the important malic-acid shuttle service, which delivers nutrients to the cells and converts malic acid into usable energy. Malic acid also helps to dispose of any excess lactic acid in the muscles.

In one study by nutritional specialist Dr Guy Abraham, of the University of California, fibromyalgia patients (fibromyalgia is a chronic pain condition) were given 6–12 tablets a day containing a magnesium and malic acid combination, each tablet consisting of 50 mg magnesium and 200 mg malic acid. After four weeks, their pain levels were halved, and after a further four weeks, they fell even more – from an initial pain score of 19.6 down to 6.5. For the next two weeks, six people were then switched to a placebo (sugar pill). Their pain scores rose from 6.5 to 21.5, the pain and fatigue worsening within 48 hours of switching to the placebo.

In another study by Dr Abraham, fibromyalgia patients were not told whether they were taking supplements or a placebo. The findings of the first study were confirmed, with the clarification that only people taking at least six magnesium and malic acid combination supplements a day showed a significant reduction in pain. To achieve the desired effect, you should take six 75 mg tablets a day (450 mg) for eight to ten months to raise your levels to normal, then two tablets a day (150 mg) to maintain the improvement.

Magnesium and malic-acid supplements may be bought separately; alternatively, they can be combined in magnesium malate. (See 'Useful addresses' for recommended manufacturers and distributors.) Consult your doctor before embarking on this treatment.

B complex vitamins

The B vitamins are known to aid the calming process and to help to detoxify hormones prior to their secretion from the body. B vitamins are also integral to the production of serotonin, an important pain-reducing, sleep-promoting hormone. B-complex supplementation is, therefore, highly recommended for people with a pain problem. Avoid taking them at night, however, as they may interfere with sleep. Follow the dosage instructions on the label.

A good antioxidant multivitamin and mineral combination

Vitamins A, C and E (known as the 'ACE' vitamins) together with vitamin D, CoQ10, selenium, zinc and manganese, work as fine antioxidants, cleaning up the harmful 'free radicals' that come from industrial pollutants, ultraviolet light leaking in through the ozone layer, car exhaust fumes, smoking, and so on. These vitamins and other substances may be purchased separately, or together in a single high-potency antioxidant supplement from specialist suppliers, and are sold under brand names such as Revenol, NutriGuard Plus or Resveratrol (see the 'Useful addresses' section for details of recommended antioxidant suppliers). The multi-antioxidant supplement will often also contain other important nutrients. Follow the dosage instructions on the label.

Omega 3 and omega 6 fatty acids

Omega 3 fatty acids were shown to be far superior to placebos in one study of people with rheumatoid arthritis by the Spanish rheumatologist Dr Rafael Ariza-Ariza. The measured expectation of future pain levels was reduced and the need for long-term anti-inflammatory drugs was decreased. Another benefit of omega 3 fatty acids is an improvement in mild to moderate depression.

Omega 6 fatty acids are another type of beneficial polyunsaturated oil. They are found in most plant-based oils, grains, poultry and eggs. Cod liver oil contains both omega 3 and omega 6 fatty acids, as does flaxseed oil and evening primrose oil. Some experts believe that a daily tablespoonful of flaxseed oil can reduce pain and inflammation.

The walnut is a good source of plant-based fatty acids. A quarter of a cup of walnuts supplies about two grams of omega 3 fatty acids – slightly more than is found in 75 mg (3 oz) of salmon.

There are no known drug or nutrient interactions associated with increased consumption of omega 3 and 6 fatty acids through foods. However, if you decide to take supplements of this nutrient, especially those containing fish oils, and you are taking a blood thinner such as warfarin or heparin, be sure to speak first with your doctor. There is no risk of fish-oil capsules being tainted with mercury and other contaminants as there is with fish.

When taking fish-oil supplements, follow the dosage instructions on the label.

Glucosamine

A type of nutrient known as an *amino sugar*, glucosamine governs the number of water-holding molecules in cartilage, and is converted to larger molecules that make up connective tissue. This nutrient is effective in reducing the effects of arthritic conditions. In a study known as the Vulvodynia Project, it successfully decreased pain and sensitivity in the muscles, ligaments and tendons of subjects with fibromyalgia.

Glucosamine is only available as a nutritional supplement and is often combined with vitamin C and the amino acid tyrosine to maximize its action. Follow the dosage instructions on the label.

5-Hydroxytryptophan (5-HTP)

Because of its ability to increase levels of serotonin, this phyto-nutrient or plant derivative is known to be very useful for fighting pain. Its other benefits include improved sleep, more energy and reduced anxiety. Follow the dosage instructions on the label.

Organic cider vinegar

Organic cider vinegar is reputed to help break down any acidic deposits in and around the joints. The suggested dosage is 1 dessertspoonful in a glass of water with a little honey to taste, three times a day.

Herbal remedies

The use of herbs is a time-honoured approach to strengthening the body and treating disease. Many studies into their efficacy have now been carried out, and in most cases their acclaimed benefits have been verified. Herbs, however, should be treated with respect. They are powerful substances with components that can trigger side effects and interact with other herbs, supplements and prescription medications. Herbs should, therefore, be taken with caution, preferably under the supervision of a trained herbalist. You should inform your doctor if you wish to start using this type of treatment. It is not advisable to use more than one herb at a time, unless you are recommended to do so by a herbalist.

White willow bark

The salicylic acid in white willow bark helps to lower prostaglandin levels in the body – prostaglandins being hormone-like compounds that can cause aches, pain and inflammation. This herb is becoming renowned for relieving acute and chronic pain, inclusive of headache, back and neck pain, muscle aches and menstrual cramps. Some people with arthritis taking white willow bark have experienced reduced swelling and inflammation. They have also benefited from increased joint mobility. However, as this herb mimics the action of aspirin, it should not be taken with non-steroidal anti-inflammatory drugs (NSAIDs). Combining it with NSAIDs would increase the risk of aspirin-related side-effects such as developing a peptic ulcer or a sensitive stomach lining.

White willow bark comes in the form of tincture, tablets, powder, dried herb tea and capsules. Choose supplements that are standardized to contain 40 mg of salicin, the active ingredient. Take the herb two or three times a day, as needed, so that you achieve a daily dose of 60–120 mg of salicin.

Ginger

Ginger is a natural spice that has been prized for its medicinal properties since ancient times by traditional healers in a diverse array of cultures. Today, many cultures use ginger to control nausea and reduce pain and inflammation. Research has confirmed its anti-inflammatory properties.

By lowering the body's level of the natural pain-invoking compounds called prostaglandins, ginger helps indirectly to relieve chronic pain, particularly when taken in the form of standardized extract. Localized pain can also respond well to ginger-oil massages. In a study of seven women with rheumatoid arthritis, reduced joint swelling and pain were reported following a course of ginger; both fresh ginger and standardized extract were used. The optimum dosage for chronic pain is now thought to be 100–300 mg of standardized extract, or 300 mg of freeze-dried herb, or 500 mg of whole-root herb, divided into three portions a day.

Cayenne

Cayenne is derived from dried hot peppers, the active ingredient being capsaicin, an oily, irritating phytochemical that can cause a burning sensation on initial contact with the skin. Applied topically, cayenne cream (also called capsaicin cream) eases pain by providing diversionary discomfort and by depleting the body's supply of substance P, a chemical compound that sends pain signals to the brain. Taken in any of its various oral forms, cayenne may help digestion and stimulate circulation. It can also relieve pain that results from diabetes-related nerve damage or the after-effects of shingles (post-herpetic neuralgia). In addition, preliminary studies indicate that cayenne cream may help to control the pain of fibromyalgia. Used under a doctor's supervision, special cayenne nasal preparations may minimize the severity of cluster headaches. Cayenne works by keeping the nerve signals responsible for perceiving itching or pain from reaching the brain.

For external use to relieve pain, it is necessary to see how sensitive your skin is to this herb and how effective it will be for you. Begin by applying a thin coating of cayenne cream or ointment to just one painful area and rub it in well. After application, thoroughly wash the area and your hands. Reactions will vary, often depending upon the formulations of different preparations: Concentrations of topical capsaicin can range from 0.025 per cent to 0.075 per cent. Initially, almost everyone feels a warm or uncomfortable burning sensation at the site of the application; this usually lingers for about 30 minutes. After a few consecutive days of applying the cream or ointment (rub it in three or four times daily), the burning effect should disappear. If, after a week, some pain relief is noticeable, treat other painful areas in the same way.

This cream should not be applied to sensitive skin, and it should never come in contact with open wounds.

Peppermint

Peppermint is a naturally occurring hybrid of spearmint and water mint. Unlike other mints, it contains menthol – a powerful therapeutic ingredient. It also contains menthone, menthyl acetate and some 40 other compounds.

Peppermint is often used with success to treat the following conditions.

Because it acts as a muscle relaxant, particularly in the digestive tract, peppermint oil can be effective for abdominal cramps and bloating that come with *irritable bowel syndrome*. Take one or two enteric-coated peppermint capsules two or three times a day between meals. Each capsule should contain 0.2 ml of oil. Some people prefer to drink peppermint tea regularly, particularly for nausea. For many, peppermint tea offers a soothing option to capsules or tinctures.

Peppermint oil can help to relieve *muscle aches and pains* in other areas. When massaged into the skin, it plays an innocuous trick on the nerves, stimulating those that produce a cool, soothing sensation and desensitizing those that pick up pain messages. Add several drops of undiluted peppermint oil to one tablespoon of a neutral oil, such as almond oil. Massage into the affected areas, up to four times a day.

To reduce the pain of a headache, some sources recommend rubbing into the forehead and temples a mixture of peppermint oil, eucalyptus oil and ethanol (ethyl alcohol).

Taking peppermint oil can help to dissolve *gallstones*. A number of studies indicate that peppermint oil may aid in reducing the size of gallstones and thus enable some to avoid surgery. Consult your doctor before using peppermint oil for this purpose. If your doctor is in agreement, follow the dosage instructions given for irritable bowel syndrome and digestive-tract problems.

Taking peppermint oil capsules can help to fight *stress*. Alternatively, the aroma of this oil when added to bath water is thought to help release tension and alleviate fatigue. Add a few drops to running bathwater to dissipate the oil.

As well as in oil form, peppermint comes as a tincture, a soft gel, an ointment, a dried herbal tea, a cream and in capsules. To brew peppermint tea, use one or two teaspoons of dried peppermint leaves to each 8 ounces of water. Pour very hot (not boiling) water over the leaves, cover the cup to prevent the volatile oil from being released and allow the mixture to steep for ten minutes. Strain and, when cool enough, drink.

Rosemary

The leaves and twigs of the rosemary plant are used for both culinary and medicinal purposes. For many years herbalists have used the plant to improve memory, relieve muscle pain and spasm, stimulate hair growth, and support the circulatory and nervous systems. It is also believed to relieve menstrual cramps and reduce kidney pain, for example, from kidney stones. Recently, rosemary has been the subject of laboratory and animal studies investigating its antibacterial properties and its potential in the prevention of cancer.

Rosemary is available as the dried whole herb, powdered extract (in capsules), tinctures, infusions and a volatile oil – the latter for external use only. The total daily intake should not exceed 4–6 g of dried herb.

The recommended dosages are as follows:

Tea: Three cups daily. Prepare using the infusion method of pouring boiling water over the herb and then steeping for three to five minutes. Use 6 g powdered herb to two cups of water. Divide into three small cups and drink over the course of the day.

Tincture (1:5): 2–4 ml three times a day.

Fluid extract (1:1 in 45 per cent alcohol): 1–2 ml three times a day
Externally, rosemary may be used as follows:

Essential oil: Place two drops in 1 tablespoonful of base oil, then massage into a painful area.

In the bath: Place 50 g herb in 1 litre of water, boil, then allow to stand for 30 minutes. Add to your bathwater.

Rosemary is generally considered safe when taken in recommended doses. However, there have been occasional reports of allergic reactions. Large quantities of rosemary leaves, because of their volatile oil content, can cause serious side-effects, including vomiting, spasms, coma and, in some cases, pulmonary oedema (fluid in the lungs).

Women who are pregnant or breastfeeding should not use rosemary in quantities larger than those normally used in cooking. An overdose of rosemary may induce a miscarriage, as it promotes uterine contractions.

Boswellia

The fragrant-smelling boswellia is a safe herb with no known drug interactions. It has properties that can help lower cholesterol and triglyceride – cholesterol being a common fatty steroid in the body and triglyceride being a common type of fat. Boswellia also works as an anti-inflammatory aid and it can be taken in combination with NSAID medication. One researcher who reviewed eleven German clinical studies into the effects of boswellia found that it had been of benefit to 260 people who did not respond well to conventional treatments. Even more impressive was the fact that some of these people were able to reduce their NSAID medication after taking boswellia for two or three months.

5
Complementary therapies and other techniques

As well as using trigger-point therapy, the Alexander Technique, exercise and good nutrition to tackle your pain problem, you may wish to try complementary and other therapies to maximize your improvement. Complementary therapies can tap into your body's energy channels to combat pain and disease. They can also boost your energy levels and provide a sense of well-being.

As you may know, the medical establishment viewed complementary therapies with scepticism for many years. Nowadays, however, there is a growing acceptance of the beneficial effects provided by these older, traditional therapies.

Complementary therapies are suitable for treating pain and disease for the following reasons:

• they are non-invasive
• they are largely free of side-effects
• they can be used in addition to long-term medication
• most are enjoyable.

Many of those who use complementary therapies report substantial benefits. Some good may be gained, however, from knowing they are doing something positive to help themselves. Different therapies appear to suit different people. Remember to inform your doctor if you wish to embark on complementary therapy.

Acupressure

Acupressure, an ancient form of oriental healing, is directly descended from acupuncture (see page 93). The technique is a way of accessing and releasing blocked or congested energy centres in the body. However, instead of using needles, pressure is applied with the thumb, fingertip or palm of the hand to the relevant acupressure points. Acupressure is reported as successfully treating stress, anxiety, insomnia, digestive problems, aches and pains, headaches and migraine, menstrual problems, PMS, fatigue and much more.

According to oriental belief, the body is charged by 'chi' energy (pronounced 'chee') which travels along pathways known as 'meridians'. A meridian is not dissimilar to a river in many ways. It has a source, an end and various points along the way where debris can accumulate. Along the meridians these points act as pumping stations, allowing energy to focus before moving to the next point on the meridian. Applying pressure to one of these points has the effect either of stimulating the energy where perhaps it has become stuck or stagnant, or relieving pressure where the chi needs dispersing.

Practitioners usually use the thumb to massage the points firmly. Neither oils nor equipment is used. This technique is believed to enhance the body's own healing mechanisms and pain relief has been reported, in some cases, to be rapid. However, in chronic conditions, improvements can take longer. At some hospitals in the UK, acupressure is available as part of the physiotherapy treatment options.

Acupressure is relatively easy to learn and there are plenty of good books on the subject. Once you know where the pressure points lie, practising on your own points will help you learn this technique.

Acupuncture

Developed in China some 2,000 years ago, acupuncture has soared in popularity in the West. It generally involves using fine needles at specific points in the body, found along meridians, or energy channels (as in acupressure), to increase, decrease or unblock the flow of vital 'chi' energy to help restore the body's balance and promote better health.

Acupuncture has been used to alleviate stress, digestive disorders, insomnia, asthma and allergies. Studies have shown that treatment prompts the brain to release endorphins and encephalins (natural painkillers), boost the immune system and calm the nervous system.

Today, as well as the traditional needles, many additional forms of stimulation are used, including electricity, magnets, lasers and herbs, on some of the 2,000 acupuncture points thought to exist on the body. You may need several treatments.

In one important study in Beijing, China, 54 people with arthritic disease were given acupuncture (warm needling in this case) using

Zhuifengsu, a Chinese herb. As a consequence, every patient reported a decrease in their pain. In another study in Russia of auriculo-electropuncture (AEP, or treatment of acupuncture points on the ear) all 16 people with arthritis felt better after treatment. Indeed, their blood samples showed 'statistically significant' improvement.

Bioelectromagnetics

Bioelectromagnetics is the study of how living organisms – all of which produce electrical currents – interact with magnetic fields. The electrical currents within our bodies are capable of creating magnetic fields that extend outside our bodies, and these fields can be influenced by external magnetic forces. In fact, specific external magnetism can actually produce physical and behavioural changes.

As a pain reliever, external magnetism is becoming more widely used, and much experimentation is currently under way. Electromagnetic machinery is even becoming a regular part of NHS treatment. The machinery creates a pulsed magnetic field that is used to aid the recovery of bone fractures, tendon and ligament tears, muscle injuries, and similar injuries. A small, light, comparatively inexpensive version can be purchased for easy-to-wear home use.

External magnetism in the form of a specially designed wrist appliance – worn like a wrist watch – is believed to be effective in treating aches, pains and injuries in any region of the body. As with other types of external magnetism, it is claimed that this appliance improves the ability of the blood to carry oxygen and nutrients around the body. It is also believed to speed the removal of toxins and other waste products. Various appliances are available for use on different parts of the body. (See the 'Useful addresses' section at the back of this book for outlet details.)

Note that external magnetism should not be used by anyone fitted with a heart pacemaker.

Biofeedback

Biofeedback is a treatment in which people can improve their health by using signals from their own bodies. Specialists in many fields use biofeedback to help people cope with pain.

In the late 1960s, when the term 'biofeedback' was first coined, research showed that certain involuntary actions, such as heart rate, blood pressure and brain function can be altered by tuning in to the body. For instance, many people calm anxiety by reading an interesting book. As a result, their heart stops racing and their blood pressure lowers. Later research has shown that biofeedback can help in the treatment of many diseases and painful conditions and that we have more control over so-called involuntary function than we once thought possible. Scientists are now trying to determine just how much voluntary control we can exert.

Biofeedback is now widely used to treat high and low blood pressure, paralysis, epilepsy and many other disorders – as well as pain. The technique is taught by psychiatrists, psychologists, doctors and physiotherapists.

A biofeedback specialist will normally teach people with a pain problem the following:

- a relaxation technique
- how to identify the circumstances that trigger (or worsen) their symptoms
- how to cope with events they have previously avoided because of pain
- how to change any habits that lead to increased pain
- how to set attainable goals
- how to gradually regain control of their lives.

People also need to examine their day-to-day lives to ascertain whether they are somehow contributing to their health problem. To use biofeedback properly, bad habits must be changed and, most importantly, each person must accept much of the responsibility for maintaining his or her own health.

Scientists believe that relaxation is the key to the success of this technique. A person is taught to react with a calmer frame of mind to certain stimuli – increased pain, for instance. As a result, the stress response is not triggered and adrenalin is not pumped into the bloodstream. Without biofeedback training, adrenalin may be released repeatedly, causing chronic anxiety, stress, muscle tension and eventually damage to body tissues and therefore pain.

If you think you might benefit from biofeedback training, you should discuss the matter with your doctor or other healthcare professional. If you have not previously had tests, your doctor may wish to conduct them to make certain that your condition does not require conventional medical treatment first.

There are now biofeedback computer games with palm-sized pulse detectors that can end chronic stress and so reduce pain. By playing the game on screen, you can learn to lower your heart rate and blood pressure, and this has the effect of decreasing anxiety and stress. (See the 'Useful addresses' section at the back of this book for details of where to purchase such games.) If you think that anxiety and stress play a large part in exacerbating your pain, you may want to try one of these games.

Homeopathy

The homeopathic belief is that the whole make-up of a person determines the disorders to which he or she is prone, and the symptoms likely to occur. After a thorough consultation, a homeopath will offer a remedy compatible with your symptoms as well as with your temperament and characteristics. Consequently, two individuals with the same disorder may be offered entirely different remedies.

You may want to visit a homeopath if you have a health problem that is not getting better or you are constantly swapping one set of symptoms for another. Unfortunately, it is a common misconception that you can just pop along to your local chemist, look up your particular complaint on the homeopathic remedy chart, and begin taking the remedy. If only it were that simple! Homeopathic training takes several years, and a lot of knowledge and experience is required before practitioners can decide on correct remedies. And, as I mentioned earlier, what works for one person may not work for another. An individual consultation is likely to be most effective.

Hydrotherapy

In 400 BC, Hippocrates alleged that bathing was useful for a variety of conditions, and pain was high on his list. A long soak in a hot bath is profoundly relaxing. It also has a calming effect on the central nervous system. Even more soothing, surprisingly, is a long soak in a bath as close as possible to body temperature (36.1° C). For best results, the water should cover your shoulders – and the longer you are immersed, the better you should feel. For comfort, place a folded towel beneath your head. The water should provide adequate support, though, as a body in water weighs only a quarter of its normal weight. Keep the temperature of the water as constant as possible by regularly topping up from the hot tap.

You may be interested to know that heart size increases by 30 per cent within six seconds of immersion in warm water, cardiac output increases by 34 per cent, blood pressure remains steady and changes within the sympathetic nervous system mean that there is a decreased perception of pain.

Hypnotherapy

There is still no acceptable definition of the state of hypnosis. It is clear that those hypnotized are in an altered state of consciousness, lying somewhere between being awake and asleep. They are aware of their surroundings, yet their minds are, to a large extent, under the control of the hypnotist. People under hypnosis also seem to pass control of their actions, as well as a chunk of their thoughts, to the hypnotist. We have all seen people under hypnosis on TV, acting out a role. Hypno*therapy* is about the hypnotist using the power of hypnotism for therapeutic purposes.

By the early nineteenth century, some physicians were using hypnotism – then called 'mesmerism' – to perform pain-free operations. Most medical professionals were highly sceptical, believing the people had been either schooled or paid to show no pain. Not until the last two decades has hypnotism become an accepted form of therapy.

Nowadays, a hypnotherapist will take a full psychological and physiological history of each patient, and will then slowly talk the patient into a trance state. The therapist can either use direct suggestion – indicating that the patient's pain, for example, will notably lessen – or begin to explore the root cause of any tension, anxiety or depression.

Hypnotherapists have found that when, in chronic pain conditions, the level of tension is lowered, many of the physical symptoms are also greatly reduced. Some experts in the field believe that the main purpose of hypnotherapy is to aid relaxation, reduce tension, and increase confidence and the ability to cope with problems. In one study into the effects of hypnotherapy on arthritic conditions, levels of beta-endorphin, epinephrine, norepinephrine, dopamine and serotonin were measured in 19 people before and after hypnosis. Following the therapy there were clinically and statistically significant decreases in pain, anxiety and depression, and increases in the endorphins that have a beneficial effect on the immune system. The conclusion was that hypnotherapy may well play an important role in easing arthritic conditions.

One common fear is that the therapist may, while the patient is in a trance state, implant dangerous suggestions, or extract improper personal information. I can only say that people can come out of the trance at any time, particularly if they are asked to do or say anything they would not even contemplate when awake. Malpractice would have to be brought to light only once to ruin the therapist's career. You may prefer to visit a hypnotherapist recommended by your doctor.

Relaxation and meditation

Deep-breathing exercises are excellent for achieving and maintaining overall health, and can be invaluable in reducing pain. Meditation has been shown in research to help to normalize blood pressure and boost the immune system, both of which are of great benefit to people with a pain problem.

Deep breathing

In normal breathing, we take oxygen from the atmosphere down into our lungs. The diaphragm contracts and air is pulled into the chest cavity. When we breathe out, we expel carbon dioxide and other waste gases back into the atmosphere. However, when we are stressed or upset, we tend to use the rib muscles to expand the chest. We breathe more quickly, sucking in shallowly. This is good in a crisis as it allows us to obtain the optimum amount of oxygen in the shortest possible time, providing our bodies with the extra power needed to handle the emergency. Some people do tend to get stuck in chest-breathing mode, though. Not only is long-term shallow breathing detrimental to our physical and emotional health; it can also lead to hyperventilation, panic attacks, chest pains, dizziness and gastro-intestinal problems.

To test your breathing, ask yourself:

* How fast are you breathing as you are reading this?
* Are you pausing between breaths?
* Are you breathing with your chest or with your diaphragm?

A breathing exercise

The following deep-breathing exercise should, ideally, be performed daily:

* Make yourself comfortable in a warm room where you know you will be alone for at least half an hour.
* Close your eyes and try to relax.
* Gradually slow down your breathing, inhaling and exhaling as evenly as possible.
* Place one hand on your chest and the other on your abdomen, just below your rib-cage.
* As you inhale, allow your abdomen to swell upward. (Your chest should barely move.)
* As you exhale, let your abdomen flatten.

Give yourself a few minutes to get into a smooth, easy rhythm. As worries and distractions arise, don't hang on to them. Wait calmly for them to float out of your mind – then focus once more on your breathing.

When you feel ready to end the exercise, open your eyes. Allow yourself time to become alert before rolling on to one side and getting up. With practice, you will begin breathing with your diaphragm quite naturally, and in times of stress you should be able to correct your breathing without too much effort.

A relaxation exercise

Relaxation is one of the forgotten skills in today's hectic world. The following exercise is perhaps the easiest:

* Make yourself comfortable in a place where you will not be disturbed. (Listening to restful music may help you to relax.)

99

- Begin to slow down your breathing, inhaling through your nose to a count of two.
- Ensuring that the abdomen pushes outwards (as explained), exhale to a count of four, five or six.

After a couple of minutes, concentrate on each part of your body in turn, starting with your right arm. Consciously relax each set of muscles, allowing the tension to flow right out. Let your arm feel heavier and heavier as every last remnant of tension seeps away. Follow this procedure with the muscles of your left arm, then the muscles of your face, your neck, your stomach, your hips, and finally your legs.

Visualization

At this point, visualization can be introduced. As you continue to breathe slowly and evenly, imagine yourself surrounded, perhaps, by lush, peaceful countryside, beside a trickling stream – or maybe on a deserted tropical beach, beneath gently swaying palm fronds, listening to the sounds of the ocean, thousands of miles from your worries and cares. Let the warm sun, the gentle breeze, the peacefulness of it all wash over you.

The tranquillity you feel at this stage can be enhanced by frequently repeating the exercise; once or twice a day is best. With time, you should be able to switch into a calm state of mind whenever you feel stressed.

Meditation

Arguably the oldest natural therapy, meditation is the simplest and most effective form of self-help. Dr Herbert Benson of Harvard Medical School has shown that meditation tends to normalize blood pressure, the pulse rate and level of stress hormones in the blood. He proved, too, that it produces changes in brainwave patterns, showing less excitability, and that it improves the white blood cell (immune) response as well as hormone response. It must therefore be considered an important and easily accessible aid to recovery for people with a pain problem.

The unusual thing about meditation is that it involves 'letting go', allowing the mind to roam freely. However, as most of us are used to trying to control our thoughts – in our work, for example – letting go is not as easy as it sounds.

It may help to know that people who regularly meditate say they have higher energy levels, require less sleep, are less anxious, and feel far 'more alive' than before they did so. Ideally, the technique should be taught by a teacher; but, as meditation is essentially performed alone, it can be learnt alone with equal success.

Meditation may, to some people, sound rather New-Age and off-beat. Isn't it worth a try, though? – especially when you can do it for free! Kick off those shoes and make yourself comfortable, somewhere where you can be alone for a while. Now follow these simple instructions:

- Close your eyes, relax, and practise the deep-breathing exercise as described above.
- Concentrate on your breathing. Try to free your mind of conscious control. Letting it roam unchecked, try to allow the deeper, more serene part of you to take over.
- After a few minutes you may wish to go further into meditation and begin mentally repeating a 'mantra' – a certain word or phrase. It should be something positive, such as 'Relax', 'I feel calm', 'I am feeling much better', or even 'I am special'.
- When you are ready to end, open your eyes and allow yourself time to adjust to the outside world before getting to your feet.

The aim of mentally repeating a mantra is to plant the positive thought into your subconscious mind. It is a form of self-hypnosis; only you alone control the messages placed there.

Mineral tissue salts

In 1880, homeopath Dr Wilhelm Schuessler discovered that disease can result from a deficiency in certain minerals, and developed the twelve original tissue-salt remedies. The natural ingredients are homeopathically prepared to a potency that is reputed to allow the cells to rebalance their salts content, which can then restore health. The tiny white tablets dissolve in the mouth, leaving a pleasant taste. Mineral tissue salts are an off-shoot of homeopathy and thus are completely safe. They can be used in conjunction with conventional medication without any side-effects.

Mineral tissue salts are reputed to be of particular benefit where the body is overly acidic, as is the case for people with chronic pain. They are also useful for treating minor illnesses from skin conditions to sinus disorders. There are more than thirty different tissue salts in all, but the most useful for people with a pain problem appear to be as below. Choose the remedy that most closely matches your symptoms:

No. 1, *Calc Fluor* (calcium fluoride). For the rejuvenation and maintenance of tissue elasticity. The indications for use are nerve pains, strained tendons and ligaments, varicose veins, deficient tooth enamel, constipation and piles.

No. 8, *Mag Phos* (magnesium phosphate). Nerve stabilizer and anti-spasmodic. The indications for use are cramps, headaches, migraine, neuralgia, muscle cramps, nervous tension, menstrual pains and flatulence.

Mineral tissue salts are available from most health food shops and chemists. Before you start a course of treatment, please read the instructions on the label.

Reflexology

Reflexology, an ancient oriental therapy, operates on the theory that the body is divided into different energy zones, which can be exploited in the prevention and treatment of any disorder.

Reflexologists have identified ten energy channels beginning in the toes and extending to the fingers and the top of the head. Each channel relates to a particular zone in the body, and to the organs in that zone. For example, the big toe relates to the head, including the brain, sinus area, neck, pituitary glands, eyes and ears. By applying pressure to the appropriate terminal in the form of a small, specialized massage, a practitioner can determine which energy pathways are blocked.

Experts in this type of manipulative therapy claim that all the organs of the body are reflected in the feet, and that massaging certain spots helps clear energy channels, and improve gland function and circulation. Reflexology is certainly relaxing. Indeed, some people fall asleep during sessions!

There is much ongoing research into the effectiveness of reflexology on painful and arthritic conditions. In one study by the Danish National Board of Health Council, where 220 people with chronic migraines and tension headaches were given reflexology for three months, 16 per cent of people reported that they were cured, 65 per cent said that the treatment had helped, and 18 per cent were unchanged. It was concluded that reflexology is able to help both tension and migraine headaches in a significant number of people.

Useful addresses

The British Pain Society
21 Portland Place
London
W1B 1PY
Tel. 020 7631 8871
Email: sandraschia@britishpainsociety.org
Fax: 020 7323 2015
Membership enquiries tel.: 020 7631 8872
Email: membership@britishpainsociety.org
Website: www.britishpainsociety.org

Pain Concern
PO Box 13256
Haddington
EH41 4YD
Tel.: 01620 822572 Monday–Friday, 9 am–5 pm; Friday evening, 6.30–7.30 pm
Fax: 01620 829138
Email: info@painconcern.org.uk
Website: www.painconcern.org.uk
Pain Concern offer a listening ear helpline and the chance to speak to another pain sufferer.

American Pain Society
4700 W. Lake Avenue
Glenview
IL 60025
USA
Tel.: (001) 847 375 4715
Fax: (001) 877 734 8758
Email: info@ampainsoc.org
Website: www.ampainsoc.org

International Stress Management Association UK
PO Box 26
South Petherton
TA13 5WY
Tel.: 07000 780430
Website: www.isma.org.uk

The Fibromyalgia Association UK
PO Box 206
Stourbridge
West Midlands
DY9 8YL
Helpline: 0870 220 1232 Monday–Friday 10am–4pm
Fax: 0870 752 5118
Email: fmauk@hotmail.com
Website: www.fibromyalgia-associationuk.org
For help, advice or to become a member of the Association and
receive information on a support group in your area.

The UK Fibromyalgia website, associated with the Fibromyalgia
Association UK
Martin Westby
UK Wellness
7 Ashbourne Road
Bournemouth
Dorset
BH5 2JS
Email: admin@ukfibromyalgia.com
Website: www.ukfibromyalgia.com
For fibromyalgia information, experts' comments and more, sign up
to receive the monthly *FaMily* magazine.

STIFF (UK)
(Support through information for fibromyalgia sufferers and their
families)
PO Box 1484
Newcastle-under-Lyme
Staffordshire
ST5 7UZ
Helpline: 01782 562366 (call-back service – leave a message and
your call will be returned) 11am–4pm weekdays

Email: stiffuk@btopenworld.com
Website: www.stiffuk.org
For information and advice on fibromyalgia. You can also access the monthly informative *News-Snips* magazine.

Arthritis Research Campaign
Copeman House
St Mary's Court
St Mary's Gate
Chesterfield
Derbyshire
S41 7TD
Tel.: 0870 850 5000 or 01246 558033
Fax: 01246 558007
Website: www.arc.org.uk
ARC funds research and provides free booklets. Please send a stamped self-addressed envelope for a full list of titles.

Arthritis Care
18 Stephenson Way
London
NW1 2HD
Helpline: 0808 800 4050
Fax: 020 7380 6505
Website: www.arthritiscare.org.uk
For help and advice on arthritis.
Tel.: 0845 600 6868 for a free copy of *Arthritis News*.

TheraCane Central
7812 NW Hampton Road
Kansas City
MO 64152
USA
Tel.: (001) 800 587 1203
Website: www.theracane.net
US supplier of massage tools (will post to the UK).

Weston's Internet Home Health
PO Box 1646
Hassocks

West Sussex
BN6 9GS
Email: sales@westons.com
Website: www.westonshealth.co.uk
UK supplier of massage tools.

Massage Central
12235 Santa Monica Boulevard
West Los Angeles
CA 90025
USA
Tel.: (001) 310 826 2209 (toll free) 888 818 2040
Website: www.mcla.com
US supplier of massage tools (will post to the UK).

The Retreat Company Store
The Manor House
Kings Norton
Leicsestershire
LE7 9BA
Tel.: 0116 259 9211
Website: www.theretreatcompany.com
UK supplier of massage tools.

Thera Cane Company
PO Box 9220
Denver
CO 80209-0220
USA
Website: www.theracane.com
To order the Thera Cane.

The Pressure Positive Company
128 Oberholtzer Road
Gilbertsville
PA 19525
USA
Tel. (001) 800 603 5107
Website: www.backtools.com
To order the Backnobber.

USEFUL ADDRESSES

The Society of Teachers of the Alexander Technique
1st Floor, Linton House
39–51 Highgate Road
London
NW5 1RS
Tel.: 0845 230 7828
Fax: 020 7482 5435
Email: office@stat.org.uk
Website: www.stat.org.uk
For information and a list of teachers in the UK, or for details of training courses, please contact the society or visit their website.

The Association for Applied Psychophysiology and Biofeedback
(formerly the Biofeedback Society of America)
10200 W. 44th Avenue
Suite 304
Wheat Ridge
CO 80033
USA
Tel.: (001) 800 477 8892 / 303 422 8436
Fax: (001) 303 422 8894
Email: aapb@resourcenter.com
Website: www.aapb.org
AAPB is the national membership association for professionals using biofeedback. AAPB holds a national meeting, offers educational programmes, produces a journal and news magazine and other biofeedback-related publications.

Society of Homeopaths
11 Brookfield
Duncan Close
Moulton Park
Northampton
NN3 6WL
Tel.: 0845 450 611
Website: www.homeopathy-soh.com

Institute of Medical and Biological Cybernetics
Website: www.bfbgames.com
Email: info@bfbgames.com
To purchase biofeedback computer games with a palm-sized pulse detector that helps you to reduce your heart rate and so reduce stress and pain.

References

Abraham, G. E., and Flechas, J. D., 'Management of fibromyalgia: rationale for the use of magnesium and malic acid', *Journal of Nutritional Medicine*, 3, 1992, 49–59

Abraham, G. E., Flechas, J. D., et al., 'Treatment of FMS with Supermalic: a randomized, double-blind, placebo-controlled crossover pilot study', *Journal of Rheumatology*, 22, 1995, 953–8

Ariza-Ariza, R., Mestanza-Peralta, M., Cardiel, M. H., Department of Immunology and Rheumatology, Instituto Nacional de la Nutrici<<o/ac>>on Salvador Zubiran, Mexico City, Mexico 'Omega-3 fatty acids in rheumatoid arthritis: an overview', *Seminars in Arthritis and Rheumatism*, 27(6), June 1998, 366–70

Hall, R. H., 'The agri-business view of soil and life', *Journal of Holistic Medicine*, 3, 1981, 157–66

Hong, C. Z., et al., 'Referred pain elicited by palpation and by needling of myofascial trigger points: a comparison', *Archives of Physical Medicine and Rehabilitation*, 78(9), 1997

Liu, X., Sun, L., Xiao, J., Yin, S., Liu, C., Li, Q., Li, H., Jin, B., General Hospital of PLA, Beijing, 'Effect of acupuncture and point-injection treatment on immunologic function in rheumatoid arthritis', *Journal of Traditional Chinese Medicine* (China), 13(3), September 1993, 174–8

National Board of Health Council, 'Headaches and reflexology treatment', Denmark, 1995

Perle, D. C., 'Clinicians Corner: myofascial trigger points', *Chiropractic Sports Medicine*, 9(3), 1995

Radin, E. L., 'Reasons for failure of L5–S1 intervertebral disc excisions'. *International Orthopaedics*, 11, 1987, 255–9

Ruchkin, I. N., and Burdeinyl, A. P., 'Auriculo-electropuncture in rheumatoid arthritis (a double-blind study)', *Terapevticheskii Arkhiv*, 59(12), 1987, 26–30

Vecchiet, L., et al., 'Latent myofascial trigger points: changes in muscular and subcutaneous pain thresholds at trigger point and target level', *Journal of Manual Medicine* 5(4), 1990

Further reading

Clair Davies, Amber Davies, and David G. Simons MD, *The Trigger-Point Therapy Workbook: Your Self-Treatment Guide for Pain Relief*, 2nd edn, New Harbinger Publications, 2004

Vicki Edgson and Ian Marber, *The Food Doctor: Healing Foods for Mind and Body*, Collins and Brown, 2004

Michael Gelb, *Body Learning: An Introduction to the Alexander Technique*, Aurum Press, 2004

Bill Gottlieb, *Alternative Cures*, Rodale Books, 2002

Patrick Holford, *The Optimum Nutrition Bible: The Book You Have to Read If You Care About Your Health*, Piatkus Books, 1998

Patrick Macdonald, *The Alexander Technique As I See It*, Alpha Press, London, 1989

Jim Robbins, *A Symphony in the Brain: The Revolution of the New Brain Wave Biofeedback*, Grove Press, 2001

Neville Shone, *Coping Successfully with Pain*, Sheldon Press, 2002

David G. Simons, Janet G. Travell, Lois S. Simons, and Barbara D. Cummings, *Travell & Simons' Myofascial Pain and Dysfunction: The Trigger Point Manual* (2-vol. set), Lippincott Williams & Wilkins, 1998

Index